AN ILLUSTRATED GUIDE
FOR THE DIABETIC CLINIC

An Illustrated Guide for the Diabetic Clinic

EMYR WYN JONES
DM FRCP
Consultant Physician and Diabetologist
Doncaster Royal Infirmary
and Montagu Hospital NHS Trust
Doncaster

Blackwell
Science

Editorial Offices:
Osney Mead, Oxford OX2 0EL
24 John Street, London WC1N 2BL
23 Ainslie Place, Edinburgh EH3 6AJ
350 Main Street, Malden
MA 02148 5018, USA
54 University Street, Carlton
Victoria 3053, Australia
10, rue Casimir Delavigne
75006 Paris, France

Other Editorial Offices:
Blackwell Wissenschafts-Verlag GmbH
Kurfürstendamm 57
10707 Berlin, Germany

Blackwell Science KK
MG Kodenmacho Building
7–10 Kodenmacho Nihombashi
Chuo-ku, Tokyo 104, Japan

First published 1998

Set by Excel Typesetters Co., Hong Kong
Printed and bound in Italy by
Vincenzo Bona s.r.l., Turin

DISTRIBUTORS

Marston Book Services Ltd
PO Box 269
Abingdon, Oxon OX14 4YN
(*Orders*: Tel: 01235 465500
Fax: 01235 465555)

USA
Blackwell Science, Inc.
Commerce Place
350 Main Street
Malden, MA 02148 5018
(*Orders*: Tel: 800 759 6102
781 388 8250
Fax: 781 388 8255)

Canada
Login Brothers Book Company
324 Saulteaux Crescent
Winnipeg, Manitoba R3J 3T2
(*Orders*: Tel: 204 224-4068)

Australia
Blackwell Science Pty Ltd
54 University Street
Carlton, Victoria 3053
(*Orders*: Tel: 3 9347 0300
Fax: 3 9347 5001)

A catalogue record for this title is available from the British Library

ISBN 0-632-05151-5

Library of Congress
Cataloging-in-publication Data

Jones, Emyr Wyn, FRCP.
An illustrated guide for the diabetic clinic/Emyr Wyn Jones.
p. cm.
Includes bibliographical references and index.
ISBN 0-632-05151-5
1. Diabetes—Atlases. I. Title.
[DNLM: 1. Diabetes Mellitus.
2. Diabetes Mellitus atlases.
WK810 J76i 1998]
RC660.J54 1998
616.4′62—dc21
DNLM/DLC
for Library of Congress 98-18405
CIP

For further information on Blackwell Science, visit our website:
www.blackwell-science.com

Contents

Diabetic neuropathies

Diabetic skin and joint disease

Diabetic miscellany

Diabetic clinic records and organisation of diabetes care

Appendices

Preface

One of my main leisure time interests is birdwatching. Many years ago I was asked about this during my interview for a place at Liverpool University Medical School. The then Dean of the Medical School, Dr Jack Leggett, asked me if I could think of any way in which my interest in birdwatching might help to make me a better doctor. I answered somewhat precociously that good powers of observation might be as important in the clinic setting as they are in the field. I have often recalled that remark in later years in the diabetic clinic when a sudden observation of a physical sign or recognition of a particular symptom pattern has helped to clarify a clinical situation.

On my bookshelves there are many excellent books on British and European Birds. Most of these are fairly weighty tomes with wordy tracts of text and with illustrations grouped together in separate sections. Whilst these books are excellent source references for reading in the quiet of the study, they are not ideal for use in the field when rapid access to clear illustration and concise descriptive text is required. The same can be said of some of the excellent major text books of diabetes which provide a wealth of information and illustration, but not in a form which is readily accessed when it might be needed most urgently—in the diabetic clinic itself.

I therefore began thinking of the need to produce a book which would serve as an on-the-spot reference for use in the diabetic clinic, to function in the same way as some of the best field guides for birdwatching, providing an immediate source of reference at the time of an observation. The format would be similar to the best birdwatching field guides, with each simple, clear illustration accompanied by a page of concise description and brief explanation. The book would be for use by doctors, nurses and other interested health professionals both senior and junior, in hospital or in primary care-based diabetic clinics, for their own reference, or to aid teaching and information sharing.

This book is the result. It is, in effect, a 'field guide' for use in the diabetic clinic. It is not meant to be a comprehensive text book covering all aspects of diabetes, and readers will no doubt consider that there are some important omissions. However, I have touched in the text on most of the clinical situations that I come across week by week in the diabetic clinic and on some of the more unusual clinical situations which can catch out the unwary. The text is illustrated in the main with photographs of examples of conditions that I have come across in my own clinical practice, and I have tried to keep the text concise and pertinent, using a 'bullet point' format to aid emphasis.

For ease of reading, the text is not referenced, but a list of suggested further reading is given on p. 133, and the appendices include a section on the organisation of diabetes care, and a section for reference on that most difficult of areas—the various types of insulins and tablets available for treatment of people with diabetes.

Acknowledgements

The encouragement (and the word-processing skills!) of my wife, Patricia, made this whole enterprise easier, and I am grateful to her and to our four children, Anne-Mair, Rhiannon, Sioned and Dafydd for all their love and support.

Mr Garry Swann in the Department of Medical Photography and Media Services at Doncaster Royal Infirmary provided valuable technical help and expertise and I am grateful to him and to the staff of the department, especially Mr Nick Exley, for the high quality photographs which illustrate this book. I also thank Dr John Finbow, Medical Director at Doncaster Royal and Montagu Hospital NHS Trust, for his help.

My colleague, Mr Srivastava Desai, Consultant Ophthalmologist at Doncasater Royal Infirmary, kindly supplied some of the excellent photographs in the section on diabetic eye disease and I am grateful to him for this and for commenting on that part of the manuscript.

My thanks to Lynne Trenery at Setpoint Media and Marketing Communications, Jane Alexander and Peter Robinson at Bayer plc and to Edward Wates at Blackwell Science for help and encouragement at important times during the preparation of this book. Special thanks to Dr Andrew Robinson, Commissioning Editor, and Lorna Hind, Senior Production Editor, at Blackwell Science for help at various stages of production of the manuscript, and for helping to turn the dream into reality.

My teachers and mentors in diabetes were Professor Robert Tattersall and Dr Simon Allison at The Queen's Medical Centre and Dr William Jeffcoate at The City Hospital, Nottingham. I shall always be grateful to them for their wisdom and support at a crucial stage of my career in diabetes.

This book is dedicated to my parents, with love and thanks.

Diabetic eye disease

Diabetic eye disease has a significant social and economic impact. It is the single commonest cause of registered blindness in people of working age in the Western World, and the second commonest cause of blindness (after senile macular degeneration) in elderly people. In 1990, in the St Vincent Declaration, the World Health Organization (WHO) and the International Diabetes Federation (IDF) jointly set targets for reducing diabetes-related blindness by one-third.

The results of the Diabetes Control and Complications Trial (DCCT) demonstrate that maintenance of excellent glycaemic control by intensive insulin therapy can prevent the development of diabetic retinopathy (primary prevention), and retard the progression of established diabetic retinopathy (secondary prevention) in patients with Type 1 diabetes.

Trials have shown conclusively that laser photocoagulation therapy is effective for sight-threatening changes such as proliferative retinopathy and maculopathy. Patients with advanced sight-threatening diabetic retinal disease may also benefit from vitreo-retinal surgery.

The incidence of cataract (i.e. opacity of the crystalline lens of the eye) in diabetic patients in their fifties and sixties is two to three times greater than the incidence in the non-diabetic population. The treatment of choice for cataract of diabetic aetiology is surgical extraction of the diseased lens and intra-ocular prosthetic lens implantation, just as it is for those without diabetes.

Blindness due to diabetes is therefore potentially preventable.

Diabetic retinopathy is usually asymptomatic until major complications arise, because pathological changes can occur in the retina without affecting visual acuity. It is therefore imperative that effective screening for diabetic eye disease should be available, with prompt ophthalmological referral and treatment of appropriate cases in order to aim to reduce the burden of visual handicap associated with diabetes.

Visual acuity testing

- Visual acuity should be tested at each annual review and the results should be recorded and compared with the results of previous tests.
- This is done using a well-illuminated Snellen chart positioned 6 metres away from the patient. Different types of Snellen chart can be provided for subjects who are illiterate, such as the 'E' chart where the patient is required to hold a cardboard letter 'E' in a position to match that of the 'E' pointed out on the chart. There is also a chart for young children with silhouettes of animals, the child being asked to identify the animal indicated.
- The characters on a Snellen chart are designed so that at designated distances their edges subtend an angle at the eye of one degree, which is the least distance apart for two separate objects to be distinctly resolved by the normal human eye. Thus, the characters on the 6 line can be distinctly seen by a normal eye at a distance of 6 metres, whereas the characters on the 12 line can be distinctly seen by a normal eye at a distance of 12 metres, the 18 line at 18 metres . . . and so on.
- Measuring visual acuity by means of Snellen chart testing is therefore a process of comparison of the visual resolving power of the subject's eye with that of the ideal 'normal' eye. The patient is sitting 6 metres away from the chart, so this is the reference distance. For this reason the results are expressed as 6/–.
- A subject sitting 6 metres away from the chart who can only see distinctly as far as the 12 line is said to have 6/12 vision. This is a shorthand way of stating that the best resolving power of the subject's eye is such that they have to be at 6 metres' distance in order to see two separate objects which a 'normal' eye can see distinctly at 12 metres' distance. In the same way, a subject whose vision is so good that they can clearly see from 6 metres' distance the characters on the 5 line is said to have 6/5 vision, implying that the resolving power of the subject's eye is such that they can see at a distance of 6 metres two separate objects which a 'normal' eye can only see distinctly at 5 metres' distance.
- Each eye should be tested in turn with the other eye covered.

- If the visual acuity is less than 6/9 then appropriate refractive correction should be put in place, usually with the spectacles the patient normally wears for distant vision (which may not be the same as their reading glasses).
- If it is not possible to correct impaired visual acuity with spectacles then the pinhole test should be used. A pinhole in front of the eye corrects large refractive error and improves visual acuity. Provided the intervening ocular structures are healthy the pinhole test is a useful test of macular function.
- Worsening of the vision during the pinhole test in a subject with diabetes may be an indication of the presence of maculopathy—macular oedema, exudates or haemorrhage.
- If visual acuity is less than 6/12 and does not correct with appropriate lenses and/or pinhole, especially if the visual acuity has deteriorated by two lines or more on the Snellen chart since last tested, or is made worse rather than better by pinhole, early referral for specialist opinion is required, even if the macula appears relatively normal on direct fundoscopy, because maculopathy poses a significant risk of deterioration of central, distinct vision.

Diabetic eye examination

- In the diabetic clinic the eyes should be examined in a darkened room by direct ophthalmoscopy using a conventional hand-held ophthalmoscope with a good, bright light and a range of lenses from +12 to −12 dioptres.
- It is not appropriate to examine the fundi without dilating the pupils.
- There are very few real contraindications to the use of mydriatic eye drops to dilate the pupils. The risk of precipitating previously undiagnosed narrow-angle glaucoma has probably been overstated. It is advisable not to dilate the pupil in patients who have had previous cataract extraction with intra-ocular lens implantation using the older sorts of implants which were hooked to the iris and might become dislocated if the pupil were widely dilated. This problem does not occur with the newer sorts of intra-ocular lens implants.
- The best mydriatic is probably 0.5% tropicamide, which has a relatively short duration of action (about 3 hours) and probably has a greater effect on the pupillary light reflex than it does on accommodation and focusing. It is therefore more acceptable to patients than 1% or 2% tropicamide, which are slightly longer acting and less selective. However, patients with dark brown irides may need the 1% strength for adequate dilatation.
- Patients whose visual acuity is better than 6/12 (with or without distance spectacles) before mydriasis are usually safe to drive immediately after the eye examination, but patients whose acuity cannot be corrected to better than 6/12 before mydriasis should be advised not to drive until the effects of the drops have fully worn off.
- With the ophthalmoscope adjusted to 0 and held up to the examiner's eye, the patient's eyes should be viewed from arm's length. The examiner's free hand can be placed on the patient's shoulder or on the patient's brow in order to help judge the distance. The red reflex can usually be clearly seen from both the patient's eyes at this distance, unless the intervening media are obscured by opacity such as cataract or haemorrhage.

- The examiner should now move close to the eye and by selecting different power plus lenses, focus consecutively on the cornea, the anterior chamber, the lens, and through the vitreous, noting any abnormalities, and gradually using successively less powerful lenses until the retina is in focus.
- The optic disc should first be viewed, examining the colour, the presence and degree of cupping, the clarity of the disc margins and checking for the presence of disc new vessels or haemorrhage.
- The retina should then be examined systematically by following each of the major vessel bundles out from their origin in the centre of the optic disc to the periphery of the superior temporal, the inferior temporal, the superior nasal and the inferior nasal quadrants in turn, so that no part of the retina is missed.
- Abnormalities to be noted include: microaneurysms and intraretinal haemorrhages ('blots and dots'); hard 'waxy' exudates; soft exudates ('cotton-wool spots'); venous beading and reduplication; arteriolar sheathing; new vessels; pre-retinal or vitreous haemorrhage; fibrous bands and evidence of traction detachment as well as scars of previous photocoagulation therapy.
- Finally, the patient must be asked to look directly into the light of the ophthalmoscope so that the macular area can be closely examined for evidence of maculopathy.

Diabetic retinopathy

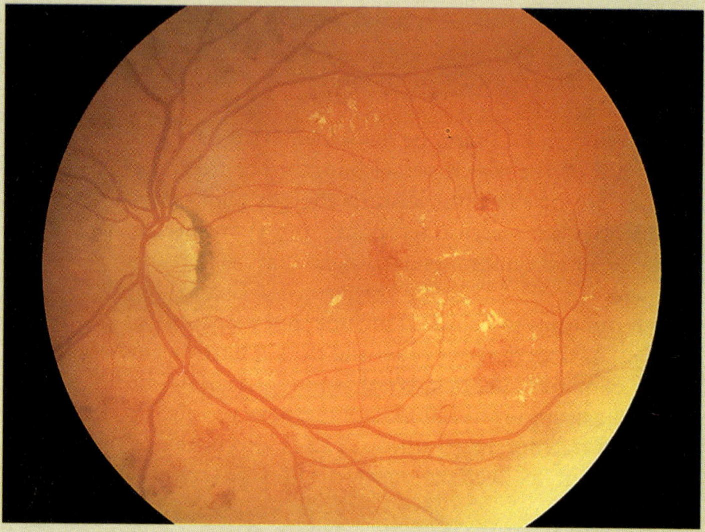

Diabetic retinopathy

- Diabetic eye disease has a significant economic and social impact. It is the commonest registered cause of blindness in people of working age in the Western World, and the second commonest cause of blindness (after senile macular degeneration) in elderly people.
- In people with Type 1 diabetes the development of retinal disease is related to duration of diabetes. People with Type 1 diabetes of less than 5 years' duration are unlikely to have any clinically detectable retinal changes, whereas over 80% of people who have been taking insulin for more than 20 years have some degree of retinopathy on examination.
- Retinal changes may be evident on examination in 5–10% of people with newly diagnosed Type 2 diabetes. This is possibly because this type of diabetes may have been present in individual patients for some considerable time before the diagnosis was made.
- Diabetic retinopathy is usually asymptomatic until major complications arise, because pathological changes can occur in the retina without affecting visual acuity.
- The DCCT demonstrated that maintenance of excellent glycaemic control by intensive insulin therapy can prevent the development of retinopathy (primary prevention) and retard the progression of established retinopathy (secondary prevention) in patients with Type 1 diabetes.
- Laser photocoagulation therapy is effective for sight-threatening changes such as proliferative retinopathy and maculopathy. Advanced sight-threatening diabetic retinal disease may benefit from vitreo-retinal surgery.
- Blindness due to diabetes is therefore potentially preventable. In 1990, in the St Vincent Declaration, the WHO and the IDF jointly set targets for reducing diabetes-related blindness by one-third.
- Effective screening for diabetic eye disease must be available, with prompt ophthalmological referral and treatment of appropriate cases to reduce the burden of visual handicap associated with diabetes.

Background diabetic retinopathy

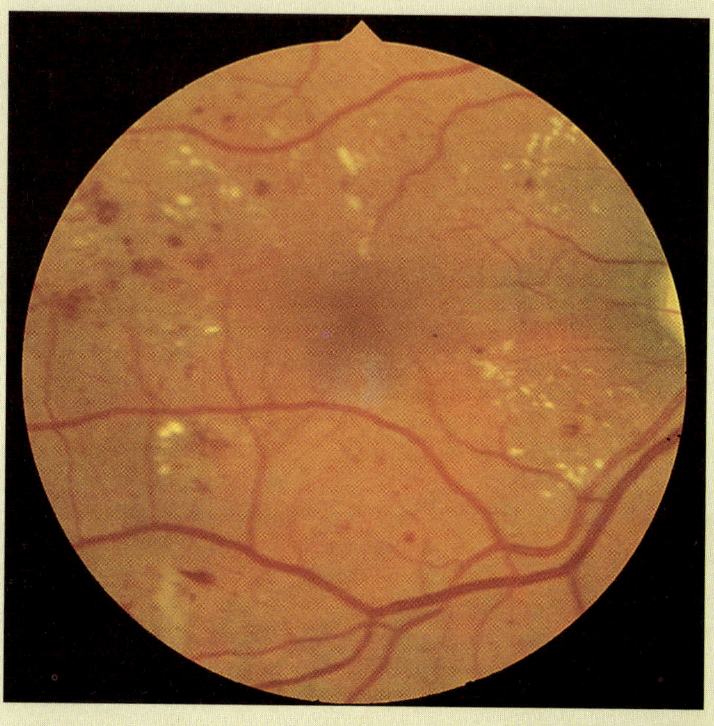

Background diabetic retinopathy

- Retinal capillaries can become damaged in diabetes, and this can cause the changes seen in background diabetic retinopathy. These consist of:
    - occasional haemorrhages and/or microaneurysms (red 'dots and blots');
    - hard exudates, not within one disc diameter of the fovea (no deterioration in visual acuity); and
    - a small number of soft exudates ('cotton-wool spots') not associated with pre-proliferative lesions.
- These lesions are not indicative of imminent development of sight-threatening diabetic retinopathy and hence do not require immediate specialist assessment.
- Close attention to glycaemic control is required, and review fundoscopy should be planned in 6–12 months' time.
- The photograph shows typical appearances of background retinopathy with 'blot' haemorrhages, microaneurysms and yellow 'waxy' hard exudates, with no encroachment of the macular area.

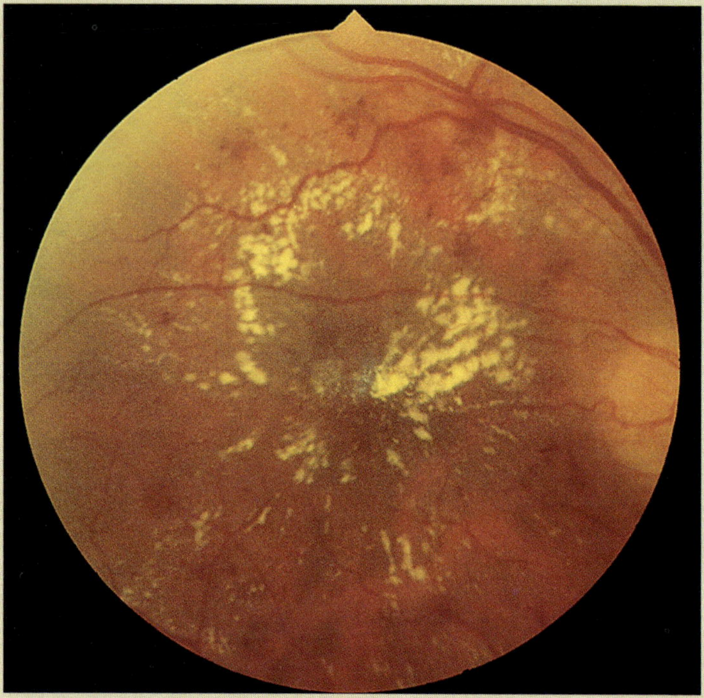

Diabetic maculopathy

- Central, distinct vision can be threatened in diabetes by maculopathy which can comprise:
  - macular oedema;
  - exudative maculopathy;
  - haemorrhagic maculopathy; or
  - a combination of macular oedema, exudative maculopathy and haemorrhagic maculopathy.
- Macular oedema is perhaps the most difficult abnormality for the inexperienced observer to identify, because the fundus may appear normal on direct ophthalmoscopy. However, visual acuity will be impaired and the pinhole test may even make the vision worse. Visual acuity that is worse than 6/12 and which is not corrected by glasses or by pinhole suggests the possibility of maculopathy, especially if the visual acuity has deteriorated significantly (more then two lines on the Snellen Chart) since last tested, or is made worse rather than better by pinhole. Early referral for specialist opinion is required, even if the macula appears relatively normal to the non-ophthalmologist.
- Damaged capillaries can leak proteinaceous material giving rise to hard exudates. If close to the macula, these can threaten central, distinct vision. Haemorrhages and/or hard exudates within one disc diameter of the macula, with or without visual loss (haemorrhagic or exudative maculopathy), require early specialist assessment.
- This retinal photograph shows waxy, yellowish, hard exudates arranged in a 'circinate ring' close to the macula (temporal to the optic disc, which can be seen to the right of the photograph). There are also haemorrhages superiorly. Laser therapy to destroy the leaking capillaries in the centre of the circinate ring might cause some regression of the exudates and prevent further progression of the advanced maculopathy which has already caused significant deterioration of central, distinct vision.

Pre-proliferative diabetic retinopathy

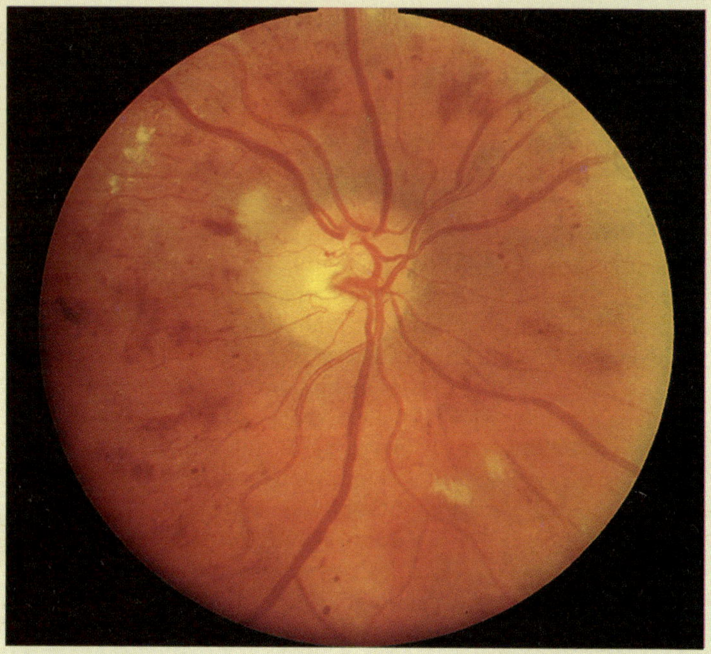

Pre-proliferative diabetic retinopathy

- Pre-proliferative changes comprise the following (in the absence of new vessels):
  - venous irregularities (beading, reduplication, loops); and/or
  - multiple haemorrhages; and/or
  - multiple 'cotton-wool spots'; and/or
  - intra-retinal microvascular abnormalities (IRMA); and/or
  - arteriolar sheathing and attenuation or obliteration of small branch arterioles.
- If three of more of the above features are present there is a 50% risk of progression to proliferation within 2 years.
- These lesions should be referred as soon as possible for specialist opinion either by an experienced physician in the hospital diabetic clinic or by the ophthalmologist.
- It is not currently clear whether photocoagulation should be given early in the development of pre-proliferative retinopathy, or deferred until characteristics suggestive of high risk develop.
- The photograph clearly demonstrates venous beading and the appearance of soft exudates or 'cotton-wool spots' as well as 'blots' and 'dots' of background retinopathy. Indeed, the process in this particular individual may have progressed beyond the pre-proliferative stage because some fine new vessels can be seen on the optic disc, indicating that this patient needs urgent referral to the ophthalmologist for consideration of laser photocoagulation therapy.

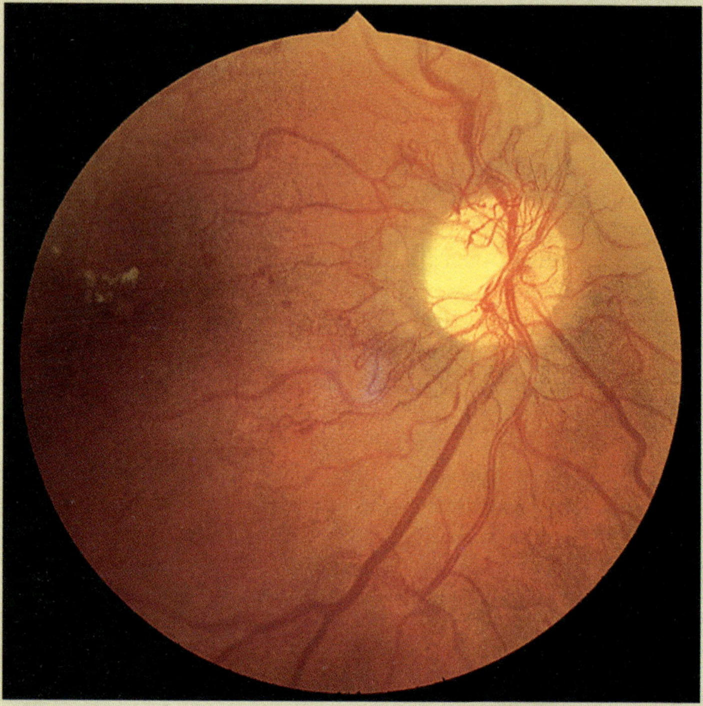

Proliferative diabetic retinopathy

- This is a serious stage of diabetic retinal disease, and if left untreated results in sight-threatening retinal and vitreous haemorrhage. New vessels on the optic disc are a sign of particularly severe retinal ischaemia and are especially prone to haemorrhage.
- The patient may have no symptoms, and therefore no awareness of the disease until haemorrhage occurs. Regular screening of patients at risk is therefore essential.
- The changes of proliferative retinopathy comprise the following:
  - new vessels on the optic disc or elsewhere in the retina;
  - pre-retinal haemorrhages; and
  - fibrous tissue.
- This is sight-threatening retinopathy. The patient has a 10–25% chance of severe visual loss within 2 years.
- Several studies have shown beyond doubt that the outcome of proliferative diabetic retinopathy is significantly improved by retinal photocoagulation. Retinal photocoagulation may reduce the risk of eventual severe visual loss by as much as 50%.
- Immediate referral to an ophthalmologist is therefore required once the changes of proliferative diabetic retinopathy have been identified.
- The photograph clearly demonstrates neovascularisation on the optic disc—the fine lacy network of new vessels growing forward from the disc which are fragile and can easily rupture, leading to sudden loss of vision through haemorrhage into the pre-retinal space or the vitreous gel.

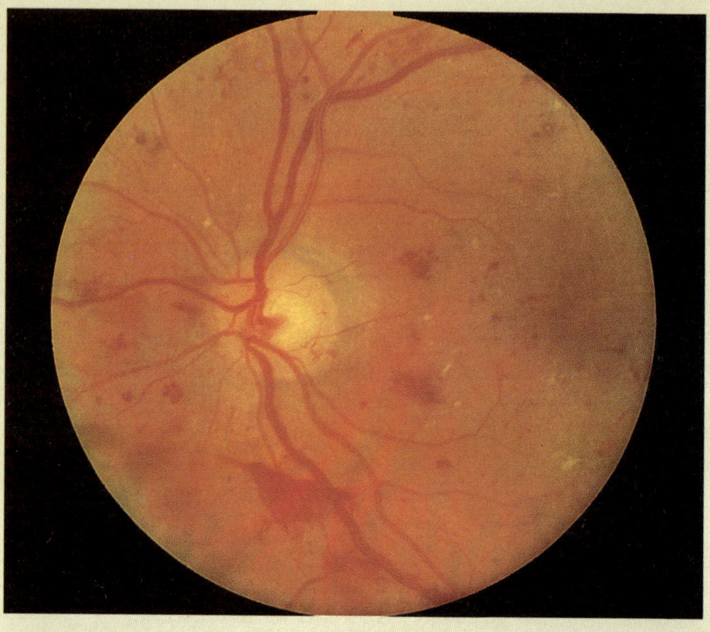

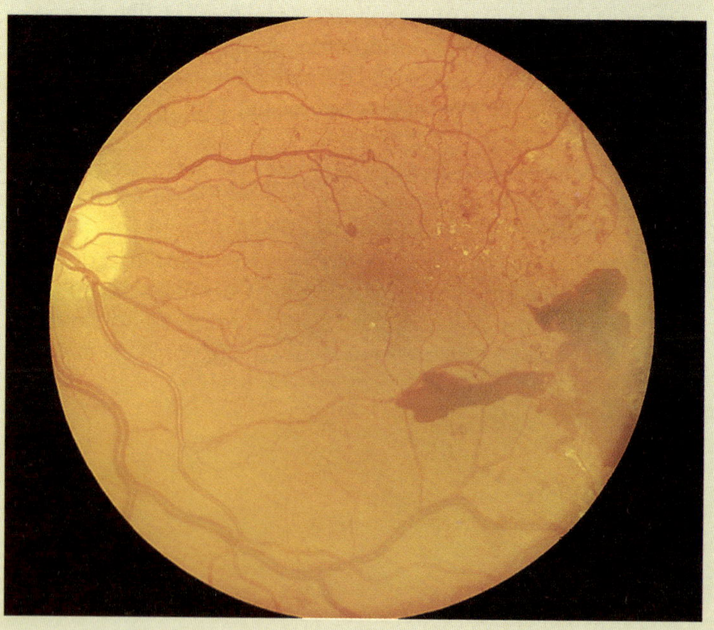

Vitreous haemorrhage and pre-retinal haemorrhage

- New vessels which form on the retina in diabetes (in response to a putative 'angiogenesis factor' elaborated by the ischaemic retina) are fragile and can break easily.
- The new vessels usually form on the surface of the retina or grow forward into the vitreous body. When the vessels break, bleeding occurs in front of the retina, either into the subhyaloid space between the retina and the vitreous body (subhyaloid or pre-retinal haemorrhage), or into the vitreous (intra-gel or vitreous haemorrhage). This can obstruct the passage of light to the retina and so cause sudden onset of partial or total loss of vision in the affected eye.
- The haemorrhage can slowly resolve as the blood is resorbed, so vision may gradually return over a period of days or weeks. However, recurrent vitreous haemorrhage can cause blindness as organisation of the haemorrhage can involve fibrosis, leading to fibrous scarring and traction retinal detachment.
- A diabetic person who has suffered from a vitreous haemorrhage requires urgent referral for an ophthalmic opinion so that an appropriate decision can be reached about retinal photocoagulation therapy or vitreous surgery, as soon as the haemorrhage has cleared sufficiently to allow reasonably clear viewing of the fundus.
- A vitreous haemorrhage or a pre-retinal haemorrhage can be visualised on fundoscopy as an obvious area of bleeding. A pre-retinal haemorrhage often has a horizontal upper edge when the patient is upright, as shown in the upper of the two photographs, where a small 'boat-shaped' haemorrhage is seen. An intra-gel vitreous haemorrhage obscures the view of the retina beyond it, as in the lower photograph.

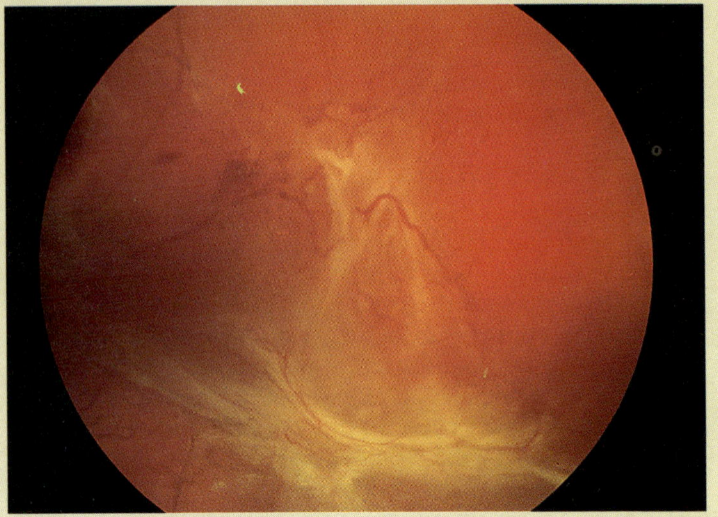

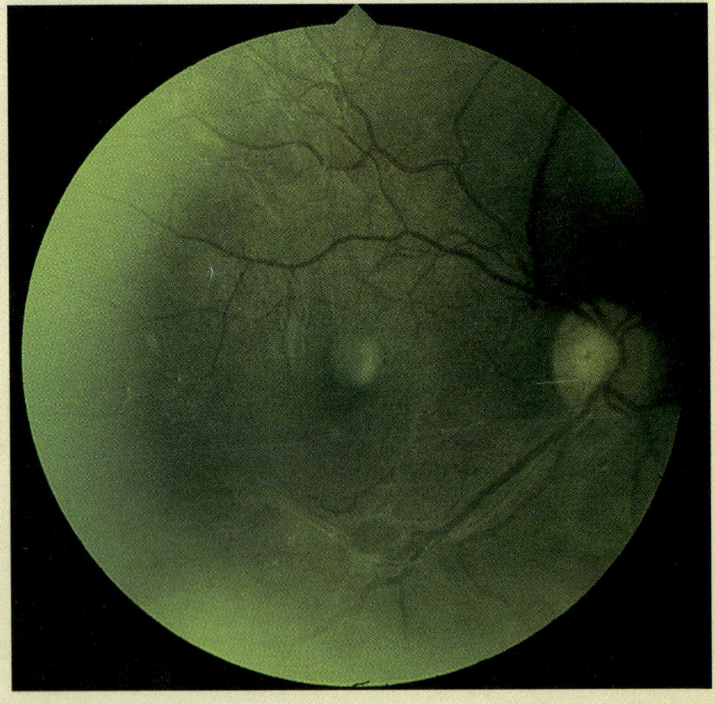

Advanced diabetic eye disease

- This is end-stage diabetic eye disease, and comprises the following:
  - vitreous haemorrhage; and/or
  - fibrous tissue; and/or
  - macular distortion due to traction by fibrous tissue; and/or
  - traction retinal detachment; and/or
  - rubeosis iridis; and/or
  - neovascular glaucoma.
- These changes represent advanced eye disease and are all potentially blinding. Urgent ophthalmological assessment is therefore required as the prognosis for sight may be improved in many cases by early vitreo-retinal surgery.
- The use of a green filter, which is provided on many hand-held ophthalmoscopes, gives a red-free image as demonstrated in the lower of the two fundus photographs opposite, and this can make it easier to visualise certain abnormalities including fine new vessels and areas of localised fibrosis.

Laser photocoagulation therapy for diabetic retinopathy

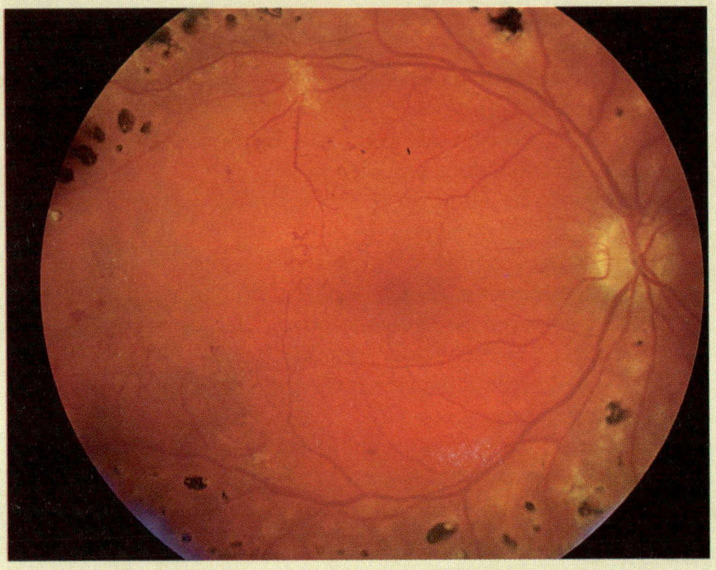

Laser photocoagulation therapy for diabetic retinopathy

- Retinal capillaries can become damaged in diabetes, and this can cause the changes seen in diabetic retinopathy.
- Damaged capillaries can leak proteinaceous material giving rise to hard exudates. If close to the macula, these can threaten central, distinct vision.
- Ischaemia, resulting from damage to the retinal capillaries, is the main cause of diabetic retinopathy.
- The ischaemic retina releases an 'angiogenesis factor' (an as yet unidentified polypeptide) in an attempt to form new vessels to overcome the ischaemia.
- The new vessels which grow as a consequence are fragile and break easily, causing haemorrhage which threatens vision.
- Blindness can result from recurrent massive haemorrhage. Fibrous scarring and retinal detachment can be other consequences.
- In pre-proliferative and proliferative retinopathy, laser photocoagulation is thought to work by causing destruction of the ischaemic areas of retina, thus reducing the production of the angiogenesis factor and reducing the stimulus to new vessel formation.
- In established exudative maculopathy, laser photocoagulation is thought to work by destroying the leaky vessels which are the cause of hard exudates.
- Photocoagulation is a destructive process which does not restore damaged vision, but simply goes some way towards preventing the progression of the disease.
- Patients having laser therapy for advanced retinopathy must be forewarned that visual field changes after treatment may affect their ability to drive.
- The photograph shows the typical round, blackened scars on the retina resulting from the multiple retinal burns inflicted during pan-retinal photocoagulation therapy, with avoidance of the macular area.

Cataract in diabetes mellitus

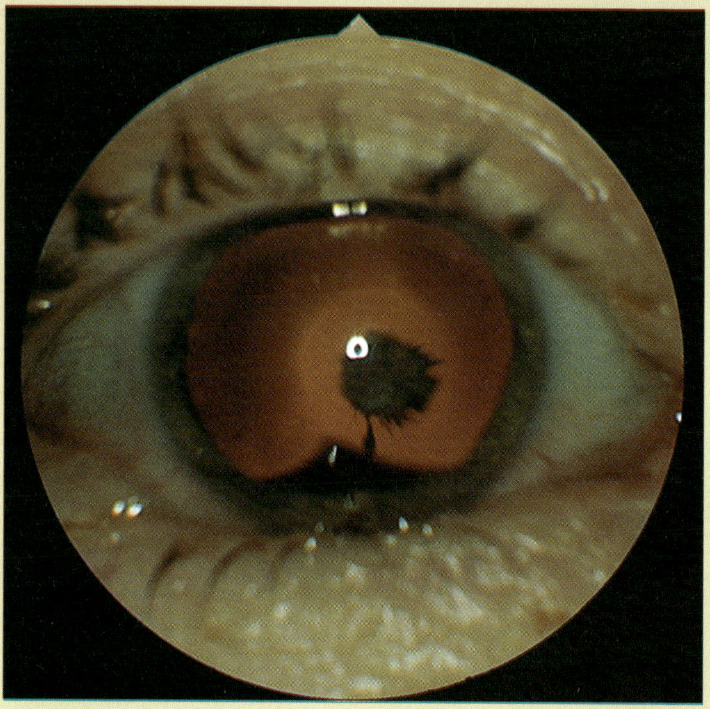

Cataract in diabetes mellitus

- Studies have shown that in diabetic patients in their fifties and sixties the incidence of cataract (i.e. opacity of the crystalline lens of the eye) is two to three times greater than the incidence in the non-diabetic population.
- The commonest variety of cataract found in association with diabetes is the so-called 'senile cataract' which may cause few or no symptoms in its early stages of development, but may progress gradually to cause significant visual impairment and even blindness.
- Some young people with Type 1 diabetes may develop an acute form of rapidly developing lens opacity known as a 'snowflake cataract'. This typically, though not invariably, follows a period of particularly poor blood sugar control, and the cataract may appear and mature in the space of a few weeks.
- Cataracts in diabetes probably arise through accumulation in the substance of the lens of osmotically active sorbitol formed in supra-normal quantities by metabolism of excess glucose through the polyol pathway. Non-enzymatic glycosylation of lens protein may also be contributory.
- Cataracts rarely may be features of other diseases or syndromes such as dystrophia myotonica which may be associated with diabetes.
- Surgical extraction of the diseased lens with intra-ocular prosthetic lens implantation is the treatment of choice for cataract of diabetic aetiology just as it is for those without diabetes.
- The photograph shows a central cataract or lens opacity obscuring full view of the fundus and interfering with the normal 'red reflex'.

Diabetic foot disease

Foot ulceration, infection and gangrene are significant causes of morbidity in the diabetic population. Admission for treatment of diabetic foot disease accounts for the use of more inpatient hospital beds than all the other complications of diabetes put together. Fifty per cent of non-traumatic lower-limb amputations occur in people with diabetes.

Diabetes is a risk factor for atherosclerosis, which is often more severe in people with diabetes than in those without, extending more distally below the knee beyond the trifurcation and leading to peripheral ischaemia.

Symmetrical, sensorimotor polyneuropathy occurs in a 'glove and stocking' distribution affecting the extremities more severely than the proximal areas, with loss of sensation leading to loss of the afferent pathway of the reflex arcs which ordinarily protect the foot from traumatic damage, and motor denervation giving rise to changes in the shape of the foot which leads to areas of callus formation over areas of abnormal pressure.

Superadded infection can cause microthrombotic occlusion of small blood vessels leading to tissue necrosis, ulceration and gangrene. Lower-limb gangrene in the seventh decade of life is fifty times more common in the diabetic population than it is in those without diabetes.

Friction from ill-fitting footwear and damage from trauma or thermal injury greatly increase the risk of foot problems in those with diabetes. The risk of foot ulceration and gangrene is also increased in those with poor foot hygiene, in smokers and in those living in poor social conditions.

Information and education about the problems of diabetic foot disease and how to prevent them may significantly reduce the risk of later amputation.

In 1990, in the St Vincent Declaration, the WHO and the IDF jointly set targets for reducing by one-half the rate of limb amputations for diabetic gangrene.

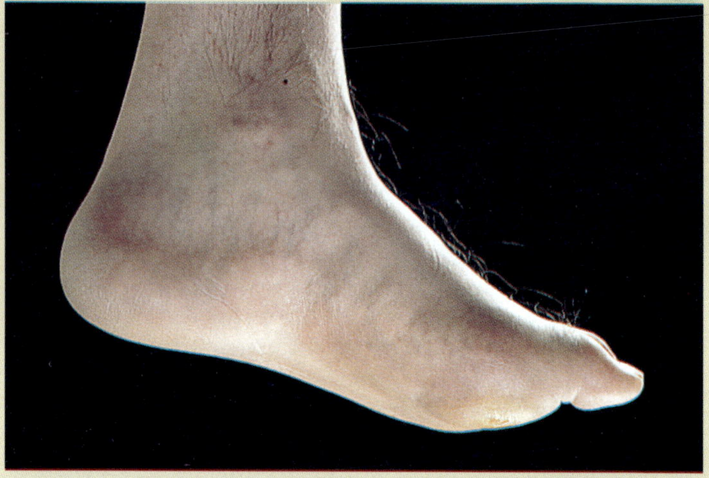

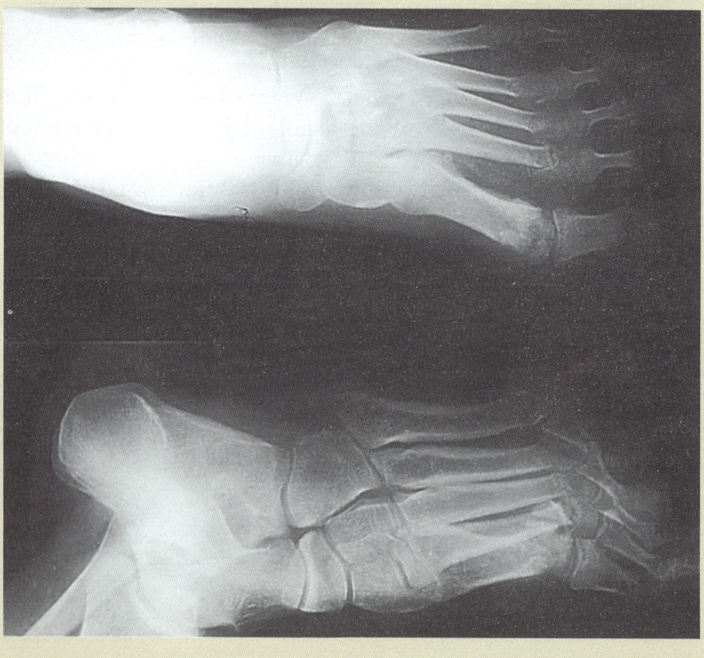

Examination of the diabetic foot

- It has been said that one of the most important acts that a doctor, nurse or chiropodist can carry out in the diabetic clinic is to persuade the patients to remove their shoes and socks!
- Careful examination for signs of neuropathy and peripheral vascular disease aids early identification of diabetic feet at risk and leads to intervention to reduce the chances of ulceration and gangrene.
- Examination should include the following.
  - Assessment of arterial perfusion including palpation of the foot pulses and possibly assessment of the brachial-ankle pressure index using an ultrasound probe.
  - Assessment of sensation to light touch, pin-prick and/or vibration. The use of instruments such as monofilaments or biothesiometers may help to quantify degrees of sensory loss.
  - Assessment of the shape of the foot, looking for clawed toes, high plantar arch with subluxation of the metatarso-phalangeal joints, bunion formation or mid-talar collapse.
  - Assessment of the skin for signs of dryness, flaking, callus, cracks, blisters, ulcers, and signs of fungal infection.
  - Inspection of the shoes, particularly the inside of the shoe for damage, rough areas or any defect that might damage the foot.
- However, even careful examination may not reveal the full extent of the problem, as in the photograph which shows the foot of a diabetic patient suffering from profound neuropathy. The foot appeared to have just a small plantar ulcer under the first metatarsal head but the presence of a degree of local redness, swelling and heat made the clinic doctor suspicious that there was more to this than met the eye, so an X-ray was requested. This showed fractures of three metatarsals and radiological evidence of osteomyelitis in the first metatarsal. Calcification was also noted in the small interdigital arteries.

Sensory neuropathy and the diabetic foot: thermal injury

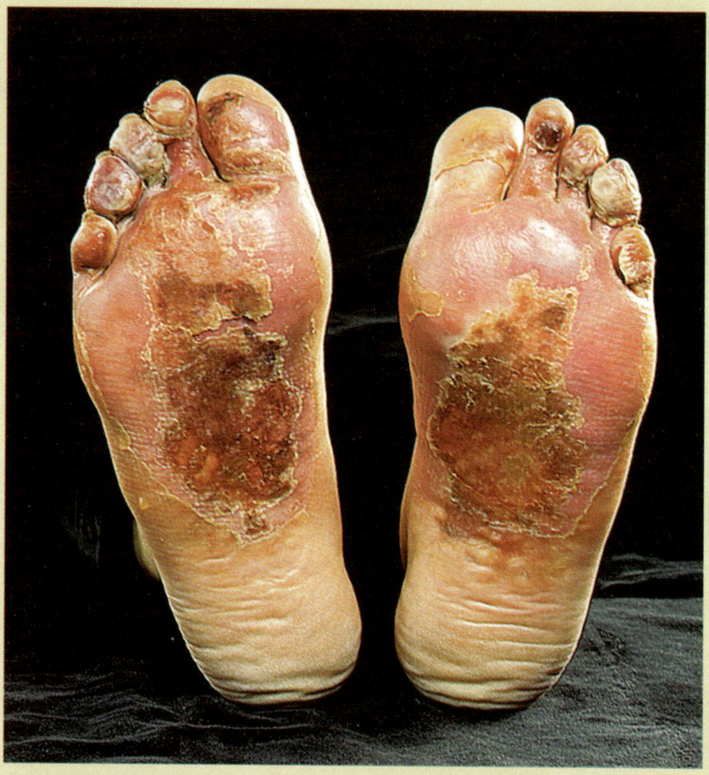

Sensory neuropathy and the diabetic foot: thermal injury

- Symmetrical diabetic peripheral neuropathy often has a predominant sensory component, with sensory diminution occurring in a 'glove and stocking' distribution—usually affecting the feet and lower legs more than the hands.
- Loss of sensation leads to loss of the afferent pathway of the reflex arcs which ordinarily protect the foot from traumatic damage. Inability properly to feel pain, abnormal pressure, friction damage or heat means that the foot is not immediately withdrawn when such noxious stimuli are present, and damage to the epidermis and then to the foot itself can occur without the patient being troubled by pain.
- The photograph shows the effects of thermal injury occurring as a result of walking on hot sand on a Mediterranean beach. The patient did not appreciate that the skin was being damaged until he saw the result—pain was not a feature.
- People who have clinical evidence of distal sensory neuropathy or who have diabetes of significant duration must be strongly advised not to walk barefoot on hot sand, not to use hot water bottles unless they are safely wrapped in a towel or special covering, not to sit with their bare feet too close to a fire or radiator and not to step into a bath of hot water until they have first checked the temperature, preferably in the time-honoured way of the mother of a baby—by dipping the elbow into the water (the hands may also be slightly insensitive to heat as a result of neuropathy).

Sensory neuropathy and the diabetic foot: punched-out plantar ulcers

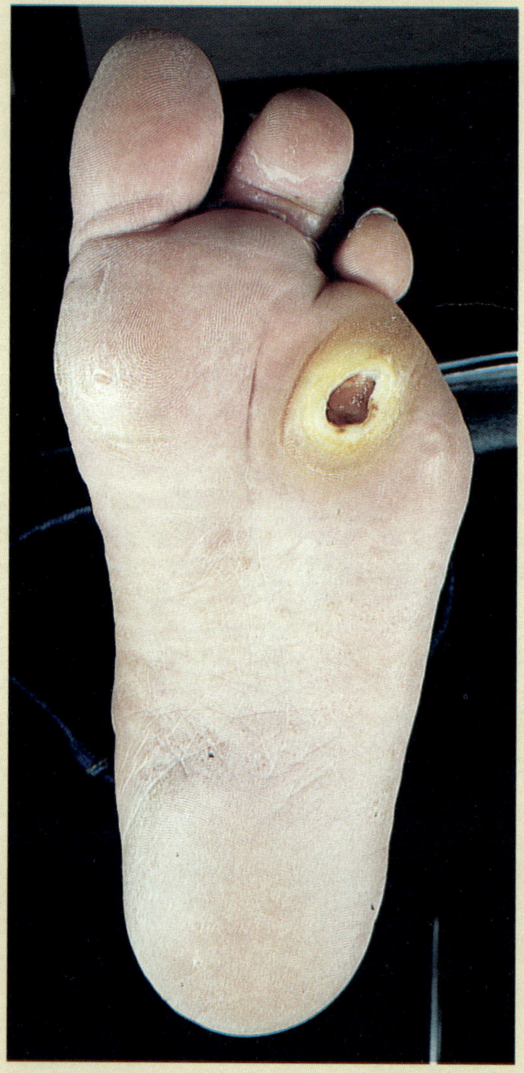

Sensory neuropathy and the diabetic foot: punched-out plantar ulcers

- Painless foot ulceration can occur because of damage from foreign objects (grit, drawing pins, etc.) in the shoe, or because of friction from ill-fitting shoes.
- Painless ulceration often occurs in areas of abnormal pressure on the sole of the foot which result from foot deformity caused by changes in the action of the intrinsic muscles of the foot caused by motor neuropathy.
- Typically, ulcers occurring in areas of abnormal pressure in the insensate diabetic foot are clean, punched-out ulcers surrounded by a rim of yellow callus. They usually occur on the sole of the foot under the metatarsal heads, often under the first metatarsal head on the ball of the foot.
- Patients with diabetic neuropathy must be advised about foot hygiene and taught to get into the habit of inspecting their feet daily to look for abrasions, blisters or damage in areas of callus which might lead to ulceration and of which they might not otherwise be aware because of lack of pain sensation.
- Patients with diabetic neuropathy must be advised to seek regular chiropody and never to try and pare their own calluses or cut their own corns for fear of causing unintentional damage to the feet.
- It is important to teach people with diabetes that footwear (shoes *and* socks) should be well fitting, made of soft materials, and inspected inside and outside regularly for areas of irregularity and for the presence of foreign bodies.
- In the photograph a typical 'punched-out' ulcer has formed in callus in an area of abnormal pressure under the third and fourth metatarsal heads, which in turn has resulted from pressure redistribution under the foot after the patient had two toes removed following earlier infections from diabetic foot ulceration.

Sensory neuropathy and the diabetic foot: diabetic osteoarthropathy (Charcot foot)

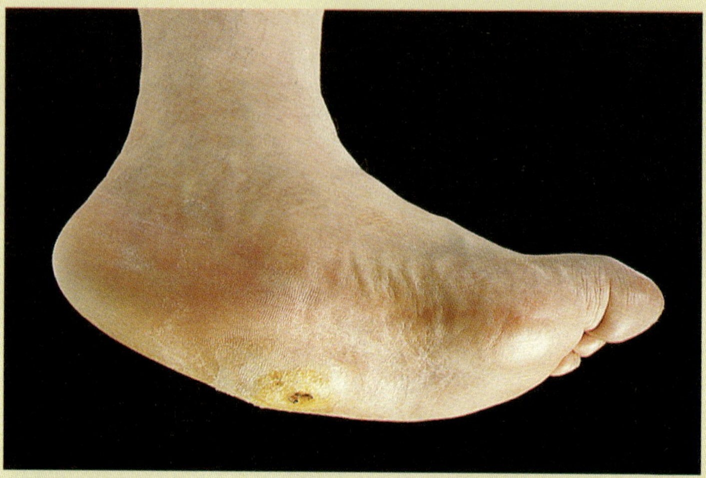

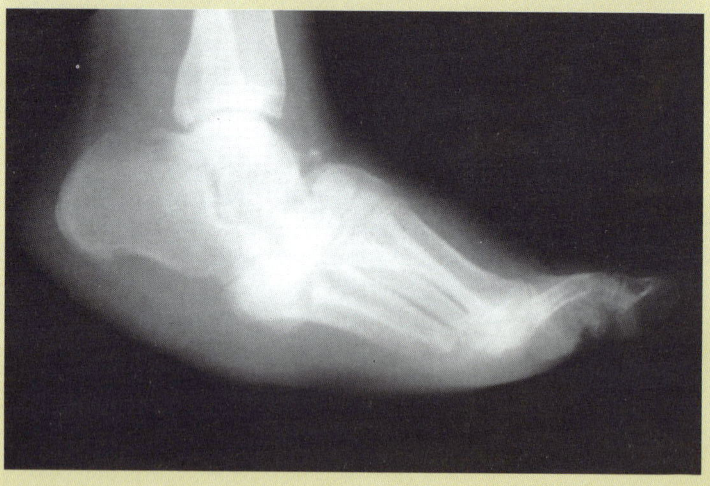

Sensory neuropathy and the diabetic foot: diabetic osteoarthropathy (Charcot foot)

- Sensory denervation of a joint from any cause may result in painless destruction of the joint with deformity, loss of joint space and peri-articular new bone formation. This is known as Charcot's arthropathy, and the resulting deformity of the foot is commonly termed a 'Charcot foot'.
- In diabetes, Charcot's arthropathy is also known as diabetic osteoarthropathy.
- Recent evidence suggests that diabetic osteoarthropathy probably often occurs as a result of stress fractures. The polyneuropathic patient fails to notice the onset of the fractures because of loss of foot sensitivity. Inflammation follows, with resorptive and osteogenic processes finally resulting in bone restoration, but with resultant deformity and functional impairment of the foot skeleton.
- The clinical picture of an acute Charcot foot is characterised by deformity in the mid foot associated with swelling, hyperthermia and redness. These appearances may mimic an acute infective process.
- In the longer term, the evidence of acute inflammation settles and chronic Charcot's arthropathy develops as a result of vigorous bone remodelling leading to hyperostosis, further joint loss and deformity. In diabetes this is most commonly evident in the talar joints, resulting in loss of the plantar arch with mid-foot deformity which is painless, although sometimes quite severe.
- The photograph shows the typical appearance of a diabetic chronic 'Charcot foot' with mid-talar deformity with loss of the plantar arch leading to the formation of an area of callus and a 'volcano ulcer' underneath the mid foot. The X-ray of the same foot shows destruction of the mid-talar joints with hyperostosis and deformity.

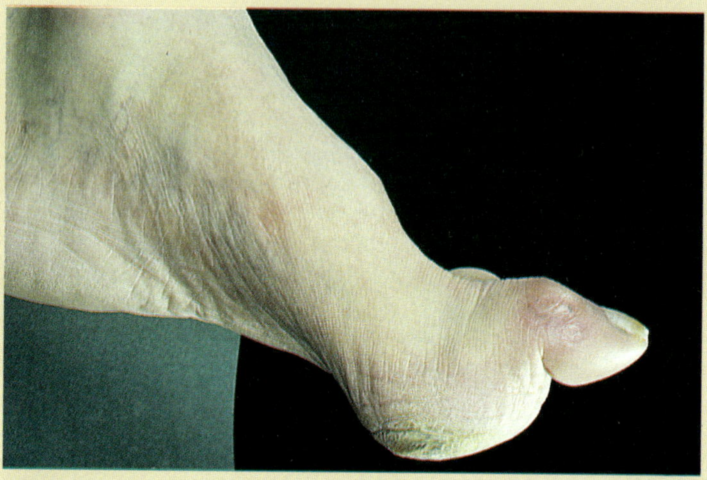

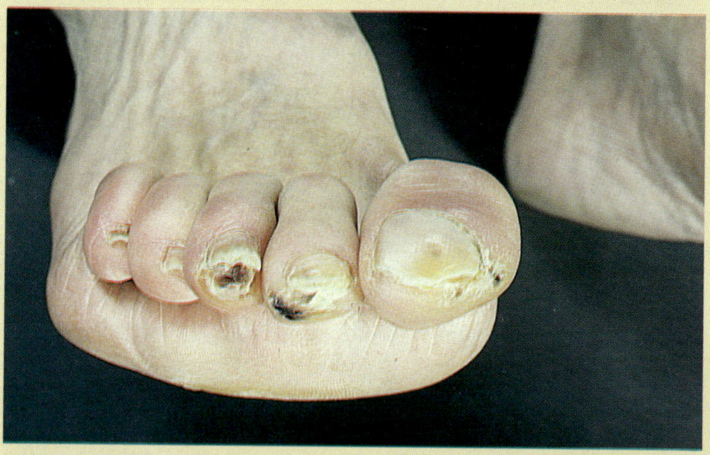

Motor neuropathies in the diabetic foot

- Symmetrical diabetic peripheral neuropathy has a motor component as well as the more commonly recognised sensory component.
- Loss of motor innervation of the small muscles of the foot leads to a disturbance in the balance of the muscles in the foot which can lead to changes in the bony architecture of the foot.
- This results in a foot with one or more of the following features:
  - a high plantar arch;
  - clawing of the toes;
  - bunion formation;
  - crowding of the toes; and
  - subluxation of the metatarso-phalangeal joints.
- The normal heel–toe motion of walking is lost. Inappropriate pressure is placed on the ball of the foot, under the metatarsal heads, leading to callus formation. The callus can crack and be the source of infection or painless ulceration.
- Callus also forms at other areas of friction such as the dorsum of the toes over the clawed interphalangeal joints where they rub against footwear, or at the tips of the toes.
- Footwear should be designed to minimise the occurrence of abnormal friction or pressure. Referral to the orthotist is often necessary to ensure provision of appropriate bespoke footwear. The shoes need to be deep and wide, made of soft materials with adequate cushioning, and no protruding seams. The positioning of a 'rocker bar' in the sole of the shoe just behind the line of the metatarsal heads may well help restore some of the normal rocking motion of the foot when walking and take pressure away from the metatarsal heads.
- The photographs show the typical appearance of a foot with a high plantar arch and callus under the ball of the foot, accompanied by clawing of the toes with friction damage causing callus to form at the tips of the toes.

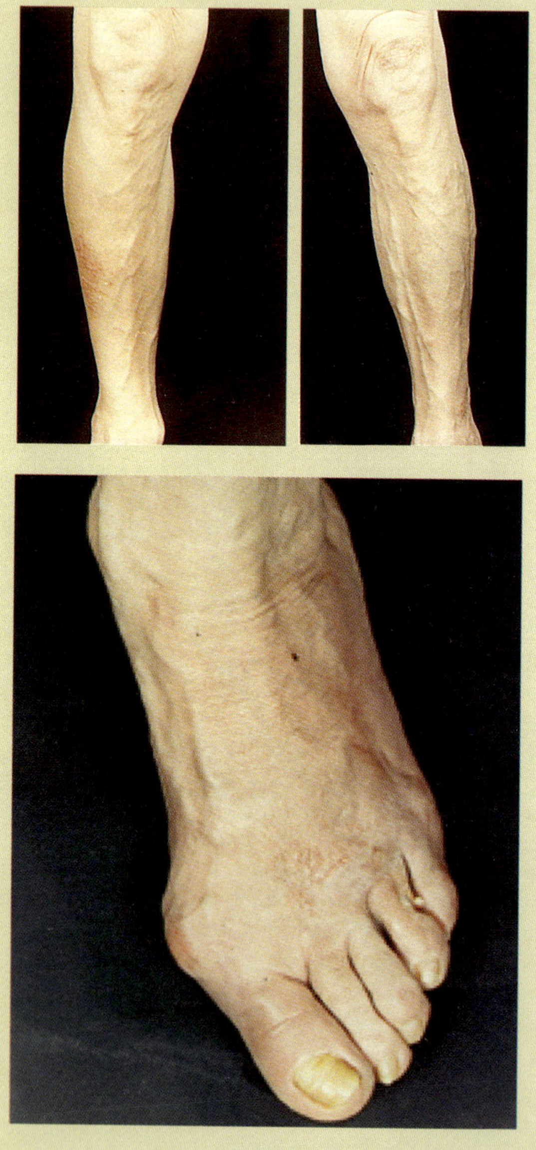

Autonomic neuropathy and the diabetic foot

- Autonomic denervation may be a significant contributor to the development of diabetic foot lesions.
- Loss of the neuronal control of sweat and other skin secretions leads to the typical dry, flaky skin which is easily traumatised. Use of moisturising lotions such as E45 cream on a regular basis may prevent this.
- Autonomic denervation can also lead to alterations in the pattern of blood flow in the leg and foot, with loss of vasomotor control leading to the opening of direct channels from the distal arterioles to the venules, thus bypassing the terminal capillary loops. The result is relative local ischaemia at the capillary level with areas of tissue hypoxia, despite the fact that blood flow into the leg and foot is good, perhaps even hyperdynamic.
- Typically, the foot affected by diabetic autonomic neuropathy is warm with dry skin. It is seemingly well perfused, with bounding pulses and dilated superficial veins which may be faintly pulsatile, reflecting the direct transmission of the arterial pulse through the arteriolar–venular shunts. There is usually associated evidence of symmetrical sensorimotor peripheral diabetic neuropathy.
- The photographs show the typical appearance of the lower legs and foot of a diabetic patient with peripheral autonomic neuropathy, demonstrating the dry, cracking skin on the dorsum of the foot and the dilated veins which were easily visible on the foot and lower leg, and which were in fact faintly pulsatile on palpation, indicating the degree of arteriolar–venular shunting.

Ulceration in a neuro-ischaemic foot

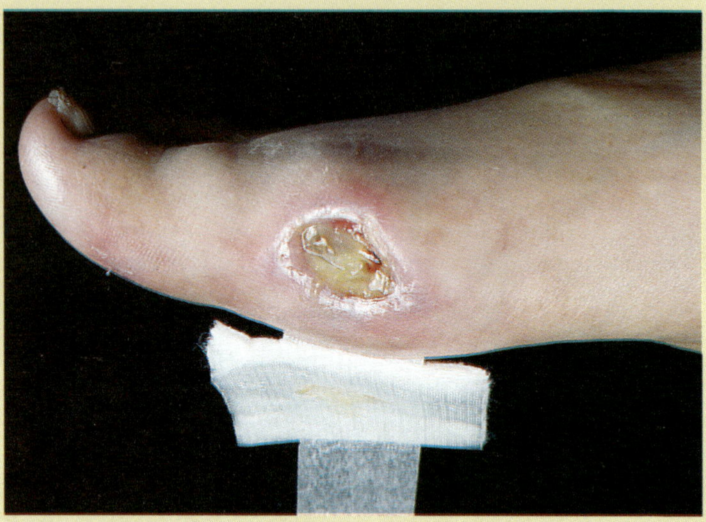

Ulceration in a neuro-ischaemic foot

- Ulceration in a diabetic foot often occurs as a consequence of the effects of both neuropathy and ischaemia.
- Typically, a shallow, clean ulcer forms over a pressure point such as a malleolus, or on the medial aspect of the first metatarso-phalangeal joint, as in the photograph.
- The foot often shows the typical shiny, red, thin skin suggestive of ischaemia.
- Peripheral pulses are absent because peripheral blood flow is reduced as a result of proximal atherosclerotic arterial narrowing.
- Sensory impairment is detectable clinically with diminution of light-touch sensation and raised vibration perception threshold.
- Despite the presence of sensory neuropathy these shallow ischaemic ulcers are often very painful.
- These ulcers are often very persistent, and may take weeks or even months to heal, even with regular dressings and care to avoid further trauma and to combat infection.
- If a proximal revascularisation procedure is posible (balloon angioplasty or bypass graft) then healing will occur much more quickly. However, it is often the case that arterial disease is too widespread in these cases to allow successful surgical intervention.
- The photograph shows a chronic, painful ulcer over the medial aspect of the first metatarsal in a patient with advanced diabetic neuropathy and arterial disease. This ulcer showed no signs of healing despite frequent and intensive attention from the footcare team, and was no smaller two and a half years after presentation, when the patient unfortunately succumbed to a myocardial infarction.

Peripheral arterial insufficiency with gangrene in a diabetic foot

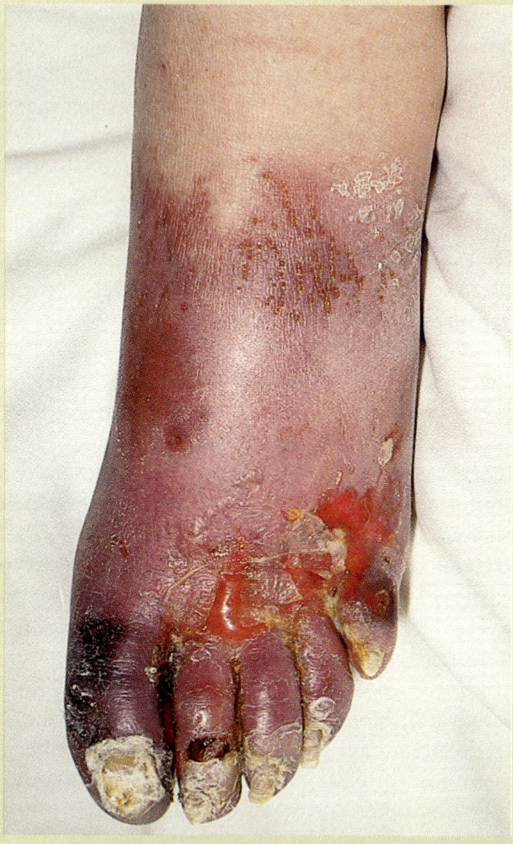

Peripheral arterial insufficiency with gangrene in a diabetic foot

- Diabetes is a risk factor for atherosclerosis, which leads to peripheral ischaemia, as well as to coronary artery insufficiency and stroke.
- Thrombo-embolic occlusion of a stenosed atheromatous artery leads to tissue infarction with non-viable ischaemic tissue rapidly becoming infected, leading to life-threatening gangrene.
- Urgent intervention with thrombolytic drugs, or with embolectomy or balloon angioplasty, or even with bypass surgery, might salvage the situation. However, this is often not possible and amputation is usually the only option.
- Arterial disease is often more severe in people with diabetes than in those without, often extending more distally, below the knee beyond the trifurcation. This makes arterial reconstruction surgery much more difficult, or even impossible.
- Smoking is a potent risk factor for arterial disease in people with diabetes as well as in those without, and should be actively discouraged.
- Lipid abnormalities occur in diabetes and may contribute to the increased risk of arterial disease, so must be actively sought and managed with appropriate dietary and pharmacological intervention.
- The photograph shows the appearance of arterial gangrene in a patient with occlusive arterial disease which was unfortunately too advanced for any effective intervention other than lower-leg amputation.

Distal dry gangrene in an ischaemic diabetic foot

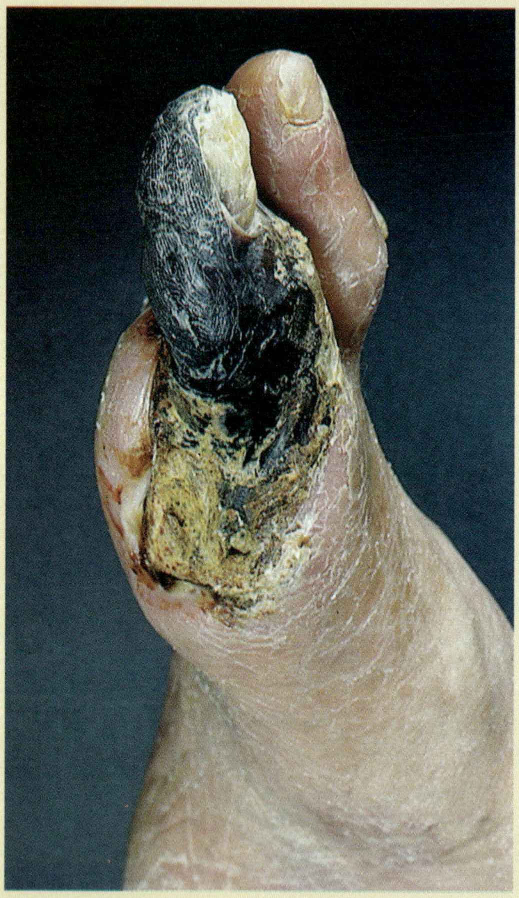

Distal dry gangrene in an ischaemic diabetic foot

- A foot which is devitalised by ischaemia and rendered insensitive by neuropathy is at risk from gangrene as a result of the effects of trauma (which may be extremely trivial), and infection which can lead to formation of microthromboses in the small distal arterioles resulting in dry gangrene of a toe or toes.
- The dead tissue often becomes mummified, becoming clearly demarcated from the adjacent viable tissue.
- The mummified toe is usually painless.
- Auto-amputation of the toe may occur, sometimes after a considerable period of time.
- The photograph shows the typical appearance of a dry, painless, non-infected great toe clearly demarcated from the rest of the foot. Regular clean dressings and good hygiene prevented the onset of infection and the patient carried on with his normal daily business for over 18 months before the toe cleanly and painlessly separated from the foot.

Fungal infection in a diabetic foot

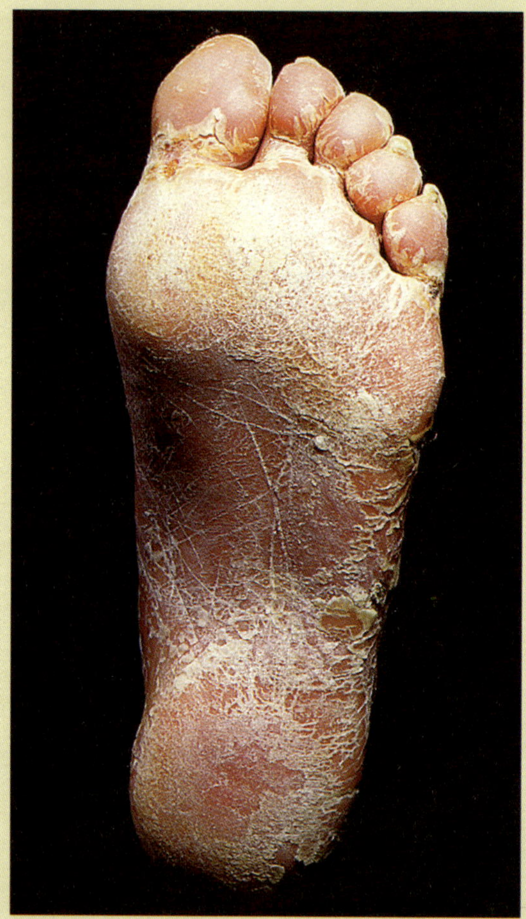

Fungal infection in a diabetic foot

- Neutrophils and monocytes from people with diabetes have been shown experimentally to have impaired phagocytosis and reduced ability to kill infecting organisms. People with diabetes are therefore more susceptible than the general population to infection by bacteria, yeasts and fungi. This increased susceptibility to infection seems to be directly related to poor glycaemic control.
- This photograph shows a severe case of fungal infection of the foot in a man with Type 2 diabetes. This failed to respond to topical antifungal agents. The cracks and crevasses in the skin of the foot acted as portals of entry for other organisms so that before systemic antifungals could be tried a bacterial infection supervened. He developed gangrene and ultimately went on to require a below-knee amputation.

Osteomyelitis in a diabetic foot

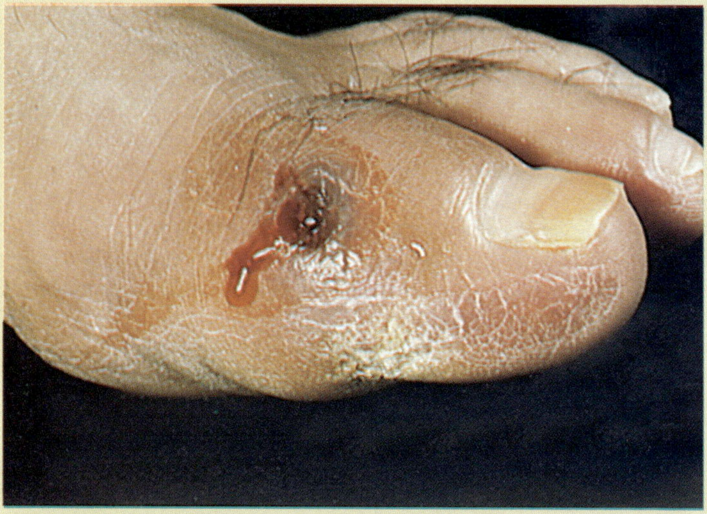

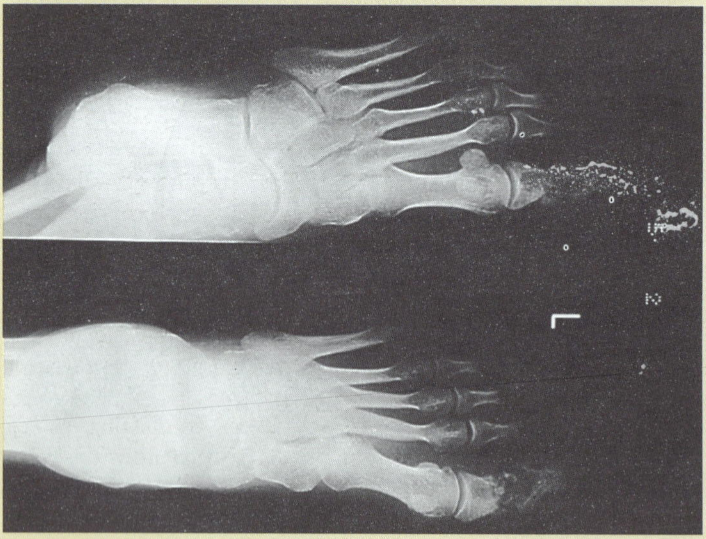

Osteomyelitis in a diabetic foot

- Osteomyelitis can occur as a result of haematogenous spread from a distant infective source, but direct infection of bone from adjacent soft-tissue sepsis is a more important mechanism in diabetes.
- Osteomyelitis possibly complicates as many as 65% of diabetic foot ulcers. If a foot ulcer can be probed to bone then osteomyelitis is almost invariably present.
- X-rays of the foot to detect osteomyelitis should be performed routinely in diabetic people with deep foot ulcers.
- If the patient is systemically well and there is no evidence of spreading infection, then osteomyelitis confined to the toes may be considered for management as an outpatient.
- Inpatient treatment is required when osteomyelitis of the metatarsals or mid-foot is suspected, when there is severe cellulitis or constitutional disturbance, when the patient is unable to comply with therapy or advice, or where there is vascular insufficiency.
- Several bacterial organisms may be implicated in the infection, including Gram-positive cocci, Gram-negative bacilli and anaerobic organisms. Antibiotic combinations must be selected which are active against all possible combinations of organisms and which have good penetration into bone even in circumstances of reduced blood flow.
- Some cases of osteomyelitis may be treated conservatively with prolonged courses of antibiotics, together with local dressings and pressure-relieving measures. Complete resolution of the infection cannot always be guaranteed even after several months of treatment.
- Most cases of osteomyelitis in the diabetic foot require surgical removal of infected tissue, and local or even major amputation is often necessary.
- The lower photograph shows an X-ray confirming osteomyelitis of the bones of the hallux in a diabetic man with severe neuropathy who had presented to the foot clinic with a relatively innocuous looking lesion of the great toe.

Medial arterial calcification (Monkeberg's calcific arteriosclerosis)

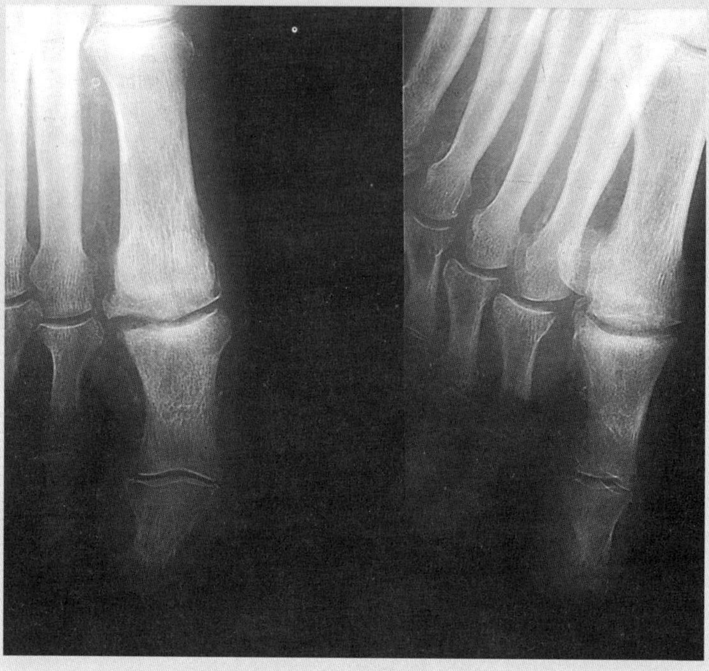

Medial arterial calcification (Monkeberg's calcific arteriosclerosis)

- Radiologically demonstrable medial arterial calcification (also known as Monkeberg's calcific arteriosclerosis) is common in diabetic subjects, although it can also sometimes be seen in patients without diabetes.
- The pathogenesis is unclear but medial arterial calcification in diabetic subjects is associated with peripheral sensorimotor and autonomic neuropathy.
- The presence of Monkeberg's calcific arteriosclerosis is a strong and independent marker of death from cardiovascular disease in diabetes.
- Interestingly, calcific aortic sclerosis and mitral annular calcification are also both commoner in people with diabetes than in those without diabetes.

Diabetic neuropathies

Different forms of diabetic neuropathy may have different aetiologies. Ischaemia resulting from occlusion of the vasa nervorum by plugs of platelets and thrombin may be the cause of the reversible syndromes such as the cranial mononeuropathies, radiculopathies and diabetic amyotrophy. Metabolic damage resulting from build-up of products of the polyol pathway, or from abnormal glycosylation of proteins may explain how chronic hyperglycaemia leads to widespread polyneuropathy, which is often chronic and irreversible. Entrapment neuropathies such as carpal tunnel syndrome and meralgia paraesthetica result from mechanical compression of peripheral nerves along their anatomical courses, and can be improved by decompression.

Chronic sensorimotor neuropathy is rarely present at diagnosis of Type 1 diabetes, but increases in frequency and severity with increasing age and duration of the diabetes. By contrast, many patients with Type 2 diabetes have evidence of significant chronic diabetic peripheral sensorimotor neuropathy at the time of diagnosis.

In people with Type 1 diabetes an acute predominantly sensory neuropathy very occasionally may be present at the onset of the diabetes. This usually resolves over a period of a few weeks as metabolic control is achieved.

Acute mononeuritis, radiculopathy and diabetic amyotrophy can occur at any time during the course of either Type 1 or Type 2 diabetes, often at times of fluctuation in stability of metabolic control. These acute neuropathic syndromes carry a good prognosis for recovery, especially if glycaemic control improves. However, full recovery may sometimes take several months.

The results of the DCCT published in the *New England Journal of Medicine* in 1993 demonstrate that maintenance of excellent glycaemic control by intensive insulin therapy in patients with Type 1 diabetes can prevent the development of diabetic sensorimotor neuropathy (primary prevention), or retard its progression when it is already established (secondary prevention).

Symmetrical sensorimotor neuropathy in diabetes mellitus

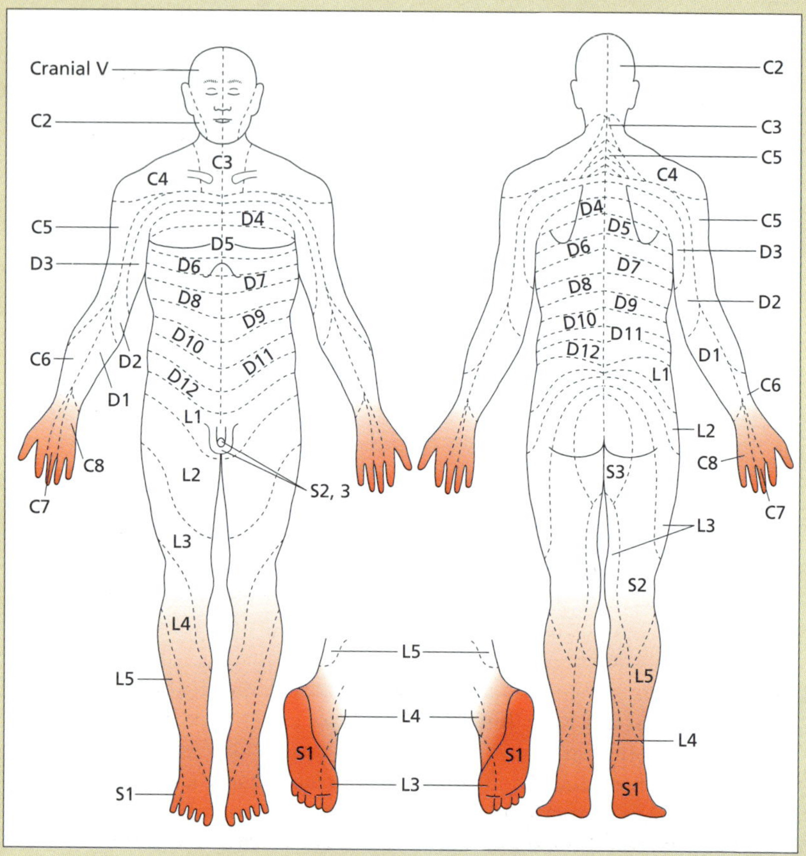

Symmetrical sensorimotor neuropathy in diabetes mellitus

- The commonest clinical neuropathic syndrome in diabetes is chronic symmetrical sensorimotor peripheral neuropathy.
- In people with Type 1 diabetes the prevalence of peripheral sensorimotor neuropathy increases with the duration of diabetes. Recently diagnosed patients with Type 1 diabetes are very unlikely to have evidence of significant peripheral neuropathy (although they may have signs of acute and reversible neuropathic syndromes related to the acute metabolic upset). On the other hand, more than half of all patients who have been taking insulin for over 20 years for Type 1 diabetes will have signs and/or symptoms of peripheral sensorimotor neuropathy
- In people with Type 2 diabetes the prevalence of peripheral symmetrical sensorimotor neuropathy is not so closely related to the duration of known diabetes. Recently diagnosed patients with Type 2 diabetes may have evidence of significant peripheral neuropathy and may even present with complications of established neuropathy such as foot ulceration.
- It affects the extremities more severely than the proximal areas. The feet and lower legs are affected before the hands.
- The neuropathic change is typically described as having a 'glove and stocking' distribution.
- Sensory function is usually affected more than motor function. The appreciation of touch, pain and temperature sensation is diminished, and vibration sensation and proprioception in the lower limbs is absent.
- Loss of motor function leads to loss of the ankle jerks, and later the knee jerks. Motor denervation of the small muscles of the foot can lead to a high plantar arch with clawing of the toes and subluxation of the metatarso-phalangeal joints leading to excess pressure under the ball of the foot when walking.
- Severe sensorimotor neuropathy can affect the hands, with sensory loss at the finger ends, and wasting of the interossei leading to weakness and clumsiness.

Cranial mononeuropathy in diabetes mellitus

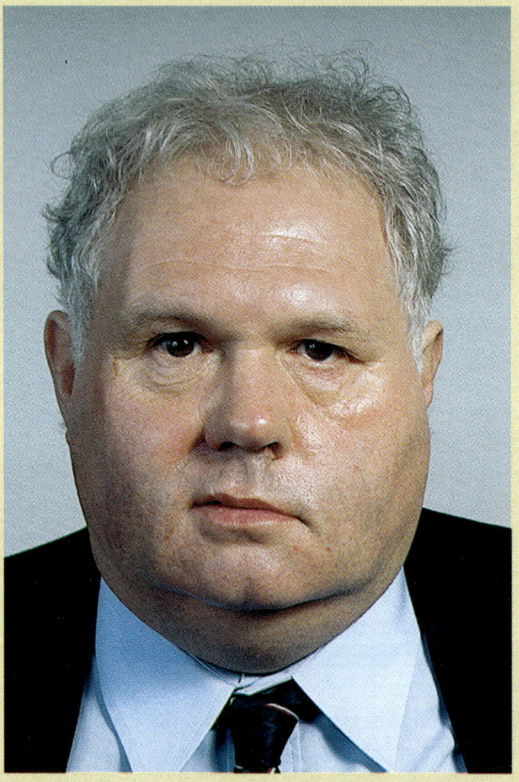

Cranial mononeuropathy in diabetes mellitus

- Isolated cranial nerve palsy is quite common in diabetes. Mononeuropathies have been described affecting each of the cranial nerves.
- A partial, pupil-sparing oculomotor (III) nerve palsy is the commonest lesion and is often accompanied by pain.
- A mild abducens (VI) nerve palsy is also common.
- A facial (VII) nerve palsy resembling Bell's palsy can also occur, as shown in the photograph.
- The cause of these isolated cranial nerve palsies is unknown, but an endoneurial vascular lesion seems likely.
- All series report a good prognosis for recovery, usually within 2–3 months.

Radiculopathy in diabetes mellitus

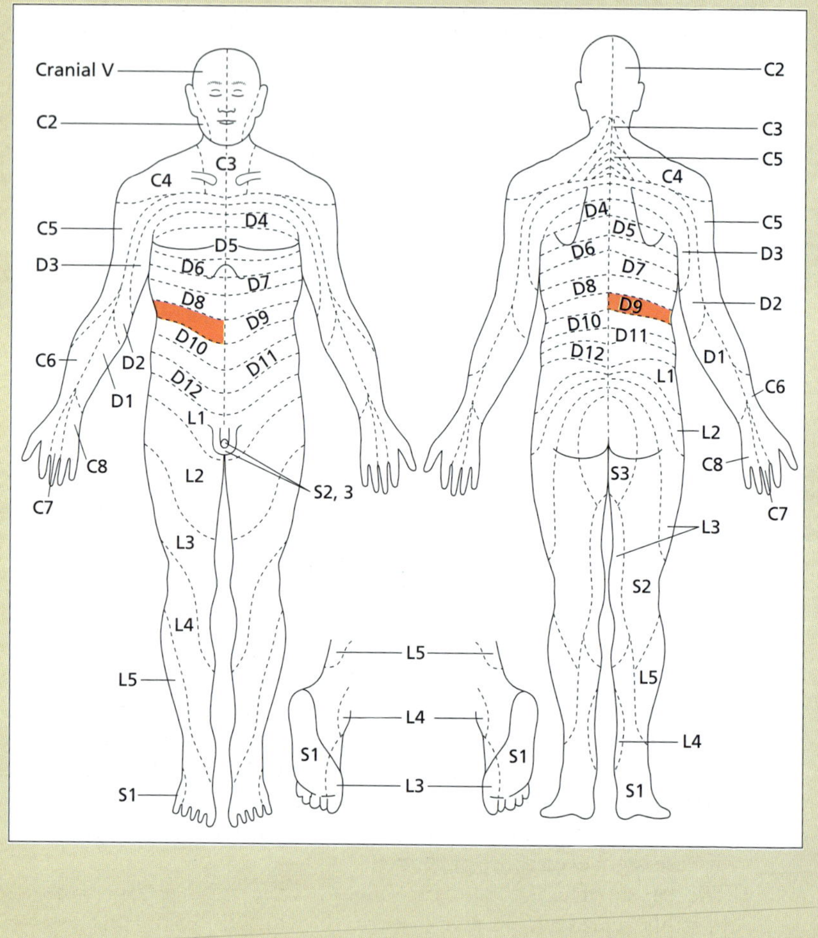

Radiculopathy in diabetes mellitus

- This usually presents with sudden onset of pain and/or dysaesthesia in the anatomical cutaneous sensory distribution of a single nerve (a dermatome).
- The symptoms may be confined to a limb, but can also commonly affect a dermatome on the trunk.
- The painful dysaesthesia of diabetic radiculopathy can sometimes be very distressing, particularly so if the patient is worried that the sudden onset of severe unaccustomed pain indicates serious underlying disease such as a heart attack.
- The abnormal cutaneous hyperaesthesia often means that the patient finds the rubbing of even light clothing very uncomfortable.
- Radiculopathy of one of the thoracic nerves innervating the anterior abdominal wall is sometimes associated with localised bulging of the abdominal wall muscles on the same side because of motor denervation and resultant abdominal muscle weakness.
- Difficulties may arise in diagnosis if the possibility of radiculopathy is not considered. For example, truncal radiculopathy affecting one of the thoracic dermatomes can be mistaken for pleuritic chest pain and lead to inappropriate radiological or isotope investigation to exclude underlying pulmonary embolic disease or other cause for pleurisy. Similarly, painful radiculopathy in the right upper abdominal area may be misdiagnosed as gall-bladder pain. The dysaesthesia typical of radiculopathy may even give a false positive Boas' sign (area of cutaneous hyperaesthesia in the right loin, associated with gall-bladder inflammation) making the diagnosis of gall-bladder disease seem even more probable.
- The cause of acute diabetic radiculopathy is uncertain but possibly represents an acute ischaemic injury to a single nerve root caused by occlusion of one of the vasa nervorum.
- The prognosis for recovery is usually excellent with gradual diminution in severity of painful dysaesthesia and return of normal sensation occurring within a matter of weeks at most.

Diabetic amyotrophy

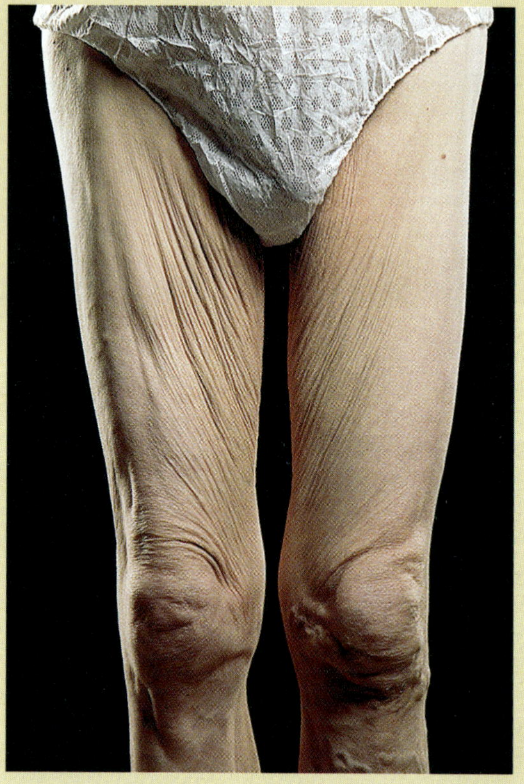

Diabetic amyotrophy

- Diabetic amyotrophy affects mainly the motor fibres and is associated with severe weakness and wasting of the proximal muscles of the legs, especially the quadriceps group, the ileopsoas muscles, and the gluteals.
- The weakness and wasting may be asymmetrical and the hamstrings and hip extensors are often relatively spared.
- The patient finds difficulty in climbing stairs or in rising from a chair without help. Sometimes walking becomes difficult or even impossible.
- The weakness and wasting is often associated with muscle tenderness and severe persistent pain, but with little or no discernible sensory loss.
- Tendon reflexes arc diminished or lost, and the plantar reflexes are sometimes equivocal or clearly extensor, raising the possibility that the underlying lesion is in the spinal cord.
- Diabetic amyotrophy often occurs in middle-aged men with existing diabetes already complicated by neuropathy, or it can occur in diabetes presenting for the first time in middle age.
- Diabetic amyotrophy may be associated with constitutional upset and severe weight loss (diabetic cachexia). Differentiation from other constitutional disorders such as occult neoplastic disease with neuropathy or myopathy may be difficult.
- There is usually gradual resolution over several months with diminishing pain and increasing muscle strength and bulk.
- The photograph shows thigh muscle wasting in a middle-aged man who had no previous history of diabetes and who had presented to the surgical team with a history of significant severe weight loss, associated with severe pain in the hips and upper thighs and profound proximal muscle weakness in the legs. A diagnosis of malignant cachexia with para-neoplastic proximal myopathy was being pursued until it was noted on dipstick testing that there was heavy glycosuria. Insulin therapy controlled his diabetes and 6 months later the weakness and pain had resolved almost completely.

Carpal tunnel syndrome and other compression neuropathies

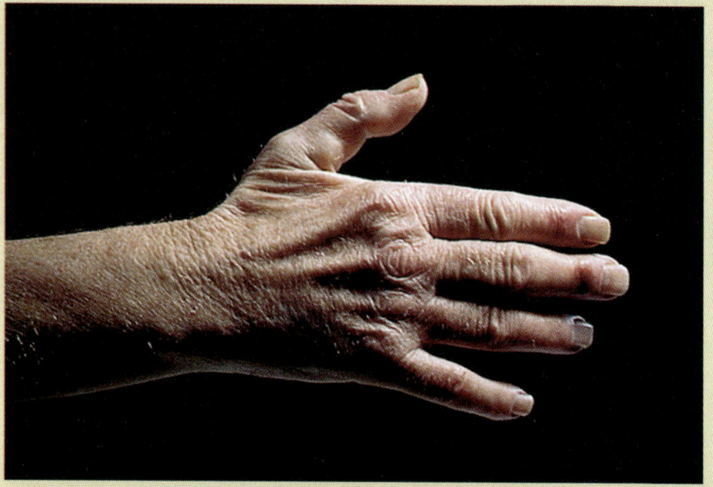

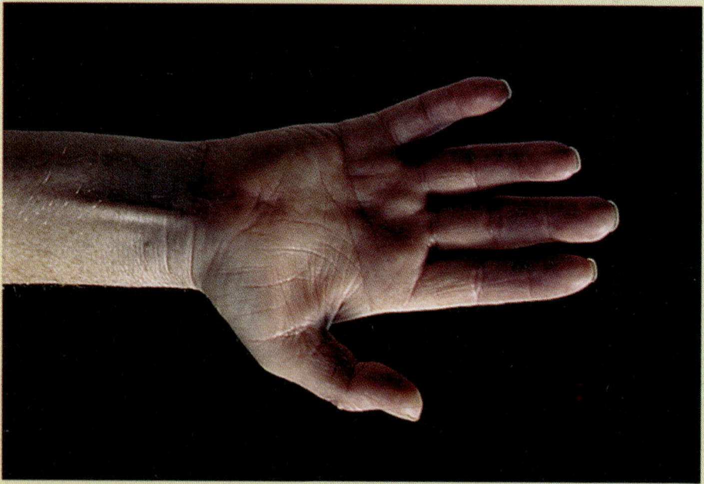

Carpal tunnel syndrome and other compression neuropathies

- Carpal tunnel syndrome (caused by compression of the median nerve as it passes through the carpal tunnel under the flexor retinaculum) is the commonest form of compression neuropathy found in diabetes.
- Symptoms include painful dysaesthesiae and sensory loss in the distribution of the median nerve in the hand (the palmar surface of the thumb and two and a half fingers—that is to the middle of the ring finger). The pain may be referred up the affected arm as far as the shoulder.
- The symptoms are often worse several hours after vigorous hand activities. In addition, the pain may be especially bad at night when sleep may be disturbed.
- There may be associated wasting of the muscles in the thenar eminence, and weakness of adduction and opposition of the thumb.
- Symptoms may be reproduced by tapping over the median nerve at the wrist (Tinel's sign), or by holding the hand palmar flexed at the wrist for 1 minute (Phalen's sign).
- Treatment consists of wrist splints, local injections of steroids in the carpal tunnel, or surgical decompression.
- The photographs show evidence of wasting of the thenar muscles and of the first two dorsal interossei in a diabetic man with recurrent carpal tunnel syndrome despite a previous surgical decompression procedure.
- A similar compression neuropathy can affect the posterior tibial nerve causing the tarsal tunnel syndrome.
- The condition known as 'meralgia paraesthetica' also occurs more commonly in people with diabetes, especially those who are obese, and particularly if the weight gain has been sudden. Compression neuropathy of the lateral cutaneous nerve of the thigh as it emerges from beneath the inguinal ligament causes painful dysaesthesia in the lateral aspect of the thigh, with corresponding sensory diminution on formal testing.

Painful diabetic peripheral neuropathy

- Many people with diabetes are troubled by unpleasant symptoms of pain or abnormal sensation in the lower legs and feet. This is often in the absence of any clinically demonstrable evidence of sensory loss or motor dysfunction, although electrophysiological tests almost always show abnormalities consistent with a diabetic sensorimotor polyneuropathy.
- Descriptions of the symptoms vary, with different individuals describing a variety of unpleasant abnormalities of sensation including 'burning', 'tingling', 'numbness', 'feeling of a tight band around the legs', 'shooting pains', 'walking on broken glass', 'walking on foam rubber' and 'walking on pebbles'.
- A frequent complaint is an intolerance of the feel of the bedclothes touching the feet at night. This symptom is known as allodynia.
- The unpleasant sensory symptoms are constant and cause considerable chronic discomfort. They are often worse at night, disrupting sleep and consequently causing daytime tiredness and depression. Because of the similarity of some of the symptoms, especially the shooting pains, to tabes dorsalis in tertiary syphilis, the syndrome is sometimes termed 'diabetic tabes'.
- There are often no obvious relieving factors and treatment is unsatisfactory at best so the problem may persist for many years.
- Improvement in glycaemic control is sometimes associated with a degree of alleviation in the symptoms of chronic painful diabetic neuropathy (although sudden, dramatic improvement in glycaemic control in previously asymptomatic individuals can also be associated with onset of an acute, usually self-limiting, painful neuropathy).
- A stepwise approach to therapy is usually adopted along the lines indicated on the facing page.

Treatment of painful diabetic neuropathy

- Simple analgesics such as paracetamol for less severe cases.
- Non-steroidal anti-inflammatory agents can be usefully combined with simple analgesics.
- Tricyclic antidepressant drugs such as imipramine and amitriptyline, starting with a small dose at night and increasing the dose depending on response and tolerance. These have been shown in double blind, controlled trials to be effective in diabetic neuropathic pain in both depressed and non-depressed patients.
- Serotonin uptake inhibiting antidepressants, such as paroxetine. Again, these have been shown in placebo-controlled trials to be effective in diabetic neuropathic pain, but they do not seem as effective as the tricyclic drugs.
- Anticonvulsant drugs can be used if antidepressants are ineffective or not tolerated. Carbamazepine has been shown in double-blind, controlled trials to be effective in diabetic neuropathic pain. It is usually started in a small dose of 100 mg b.d., building up to a larger dose, if required. Phenytoin has also been shown in placebo-controlled trials to be effective, but it does not seem as effective as carbamazepine.
- The local anaesthetic drugs lignocaine and mexilitene have both been shown in placebo-controlled trials to be effective in relieving diabetic neuropathic pain, with the response to intravenous lignocaine (5 mg/kg body weight) sometimes lasting for 2–3 weeks, and predicting the response to oral mexilitene.
- Capsaicin, a substance extracted from red chilli peppers, causes release of substance P from sensory nerve endings. It has been shown in trials to be effective in relieving diabetic neuropathic pain after repeated topical application. Local irritation and burning can, however, significantly limit its use.
- Other, less well proven therapies include the use of oral clonidine, pentoxifylline and clonazepam, as well as the local application of the surgical skin protector 'opsite dressing'.

Gustatory sweats

- This well recognised but uncommon manifestation of diabetic autonomic neuropathy results in profuse facial sweating which occurs on ingestion of food or drink. Unlike the more common unilateral sweating of Frey's syndrome which follows parotid or other head and neck surgery, diabetic gustatory sweating is bilateral and is invariably associated with autonomic and peripheral neuropathy.
- There is usually evidence of autonomic neuropathy affecting other systems, such as postural hypotension and loss of the normal respiratory variation in the pulse rate. Male patients may have complaints of erectile dysfunction or there may be a history suggestive of bladder or bowel dysfunction or of delayed gastric emptying.
- The sweating responds to the use of the oral antimuscarinic drugs such as probantheline bromide, but the side-effects of treatment are common and limiting.
- Topical 0.5% glycopyrrolate cream applied on alternate days can be useful and has no adverse effects if care is taken not to allow contact with the eyes and delicate mucous membranes.
- Gustatory sweating may be due to abnormal innervation, with intermingling of parasympathetic and secretomotor nerve fibres. However, in one diabetic patient with gustatory sweating and hypotension, anti-sympathetic ganglia antibodies have been described, suggesting the possibility that there may be an alternative mechanism.

Diabetic skin and joint disease

The term 'diabetic dermopathy' is reserved for the skin condition characterised by small, pigmented spots which appear on the anterior aspects of the shin, usually in elderly patients with long-standing diabetes, and which may progress to small, shiny, atrophic scars. It is often associated with peripheral vascular disease and/or neuropathy and may therefore be an indication of a foot at risk of ulceration and gangrene.

The skin condition known as necrobiosis lipoidica diabeticorum is a specific association of diabetes and may sometimes even herald the onset of diabetes. The histologically similar but clinically distinct condition of granuloma annulare, though associated with diabetes, can also occur in people without diabetes.

Vitiligo is a marker of the autoimmune mechanisms which are thought to be the root cause of Type 1 diabetes, and may also be associated with other organ-specific autoimmune disorders.

Bacterial and fungal infections of the skin occur more frequently in people with poorly controlled diabetes, probably because they have impaired phagocytic function of monocytes and neutrophils, and breakdown of other defence mechanisms.

Severe hypertriglyceridaemia in poorly controlled diabetes can lead to the condition of eruptive xanthomata (xanthoma diabeticorum). Triglyceride deposition in the skin leads to the formation of characteristic skin lesions which usually regress when the underlying hypertriglyceridaemia is corrected.

Long-term complications of diabetes such as vasculopathy and neuropathy probably contribute to the causation of diabetes-related skin conditions such as bullosis diabeticorum.

Non-enzymatic glycosylation of collagen and other structural proteins in the skin and soft tissues probably cause the changes of diabetic cheiroarthropathy and limited joint mobility. The same mechanisms may explain the increased prevalence of abnormalities such as periarthritis of the shoulder and Dupuytren's contracture, both of which are commoner in people with diabetes than in those without.

Necrobiosis lipoidica diabeticorum

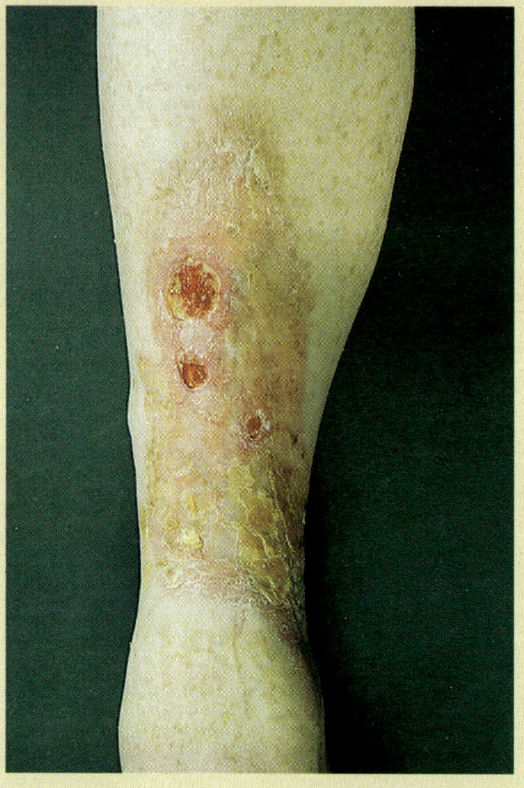

Necrobiosis lipoidica diabeticorum

- This is a skin condition occurring far more frequently in people with diabetes than in the non-diabetic population. It may sometimes predate the onset of diabetes by a significant length of time.
- It occurs in women more commonly than in men (3:1) and is unrelated to duration or type of diabetes, or to the degree of short-term or long-term control.
- Typically, the lesions appear on the shin, are usually bilateral, starting as small papules which often grow and coalesce to form large irregular plaques. These demonstrate the typical appearance of non-scaling plaques with atrophic, yellow centres, surface telangiectasia and violaceous or erythematous border (sometimes raised).
- Ulceration can occur in up to one-third of the lesions. This is shown in the accompanying photograph of an extensive area of typical necrobiosis with ulceration on the anterior shin of a patient with longstanding Type 1 diabetes.
- Uncommonly (10–15% of cases) lesions occur in areas other than the anterior shins, such as on the extensor surface of the forearms.
- Spontaneous remission can occur in up to 20% of cases.
- Treatment is disappointing. Intralesional steroid injection into the rim of the lesion may prevent progression. Topical steroids should not be used where there is significant atrophy. Cosmetic preparations may be useful to camouflage the lesions.

Granuloma annulare

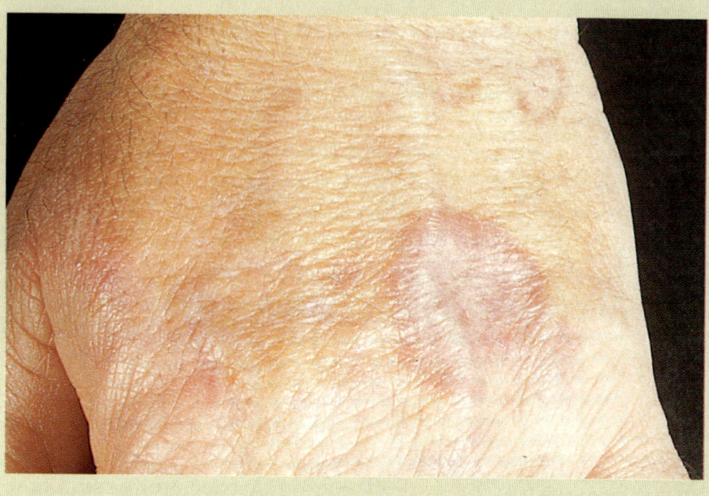

Granuloma annulare

- Although this condition is histologically similar to necrobiosis lipoidica diabeticorum, evidence for its association with diabetes is much more tenuous. Many published series indicate a weak connection, or none at all, although one retrospective series suggested an association between one form of granuloma annulare and insulin-dependent diabetes.
- Lesions consist of a ring of flesh-coloured papules, which may be solitary or multiple.
- The commonest sites are on the dorsal surfaces of the hands, wrists and feet, though sometimes lesions may occur on more proximal parts of the limbs and there is also a generalised form.
- The lesions are not usually itchy and there are no other local or generalised symptoms.
- The lesions usually resolve spontaneously in 1 or 2 years, but it can sometimes take longer and recurrences can occur.
- Topical or intralesional steroids may hasten resolution.
- Oral potassium iodide has been shown to be of benefit in some cases.
- The photograph shows a typical annular slightly raised lesion on the dorsum of the hand of a patient with Type 1 diabetes of relatively recent onset.

Bullosis diabeticorum

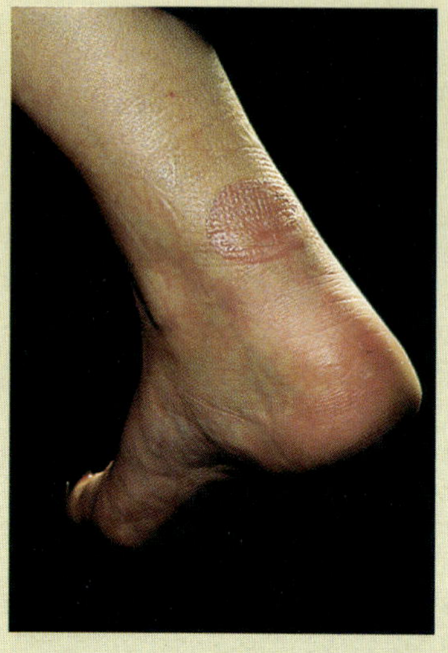

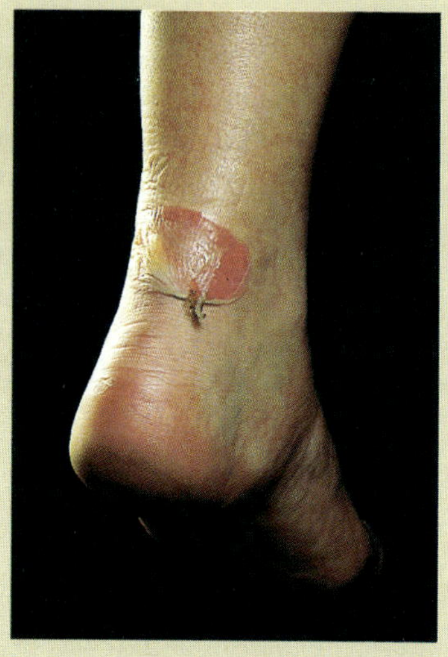

Bullosis diabeticorum

- Bullae may arise spontaneously in patients with diabetes which is longstanding, especially in those with evidence of peripheral and autonomic neuropathy.
- The bullae are intra-epidermal, arising at the epidermal–dermal junction.
- Bullae may appear on the fingers, toes, hands, feet and lower legs.
- Bullae usually arise at areas of trauma, which is often unrecognised. Even trivial trauma such as friction from clothing can give rise to large bullae.
- Sometimes the bullae appear to be symmetrically distributed, but this apparent symmetry can usually be explained by the fact that similar friction trauma is operating at both sites. The examples in the photographs demonstrate symmetrical bullae caused by friction from shoes over the Achilles tendons of both feet in a diabetic patient.
- Bullae which burst can act as portals of entry for infection. The absence of protective sensory stimuli because of the coexistence of diabetic sensory neuropathy means that the seriousness of the infection may not be recognised by the patient and serious, spreading infection such as cellulitis may result, leading to tissue destruction and even gangrene.

Vitiligo and diabetes mellitus

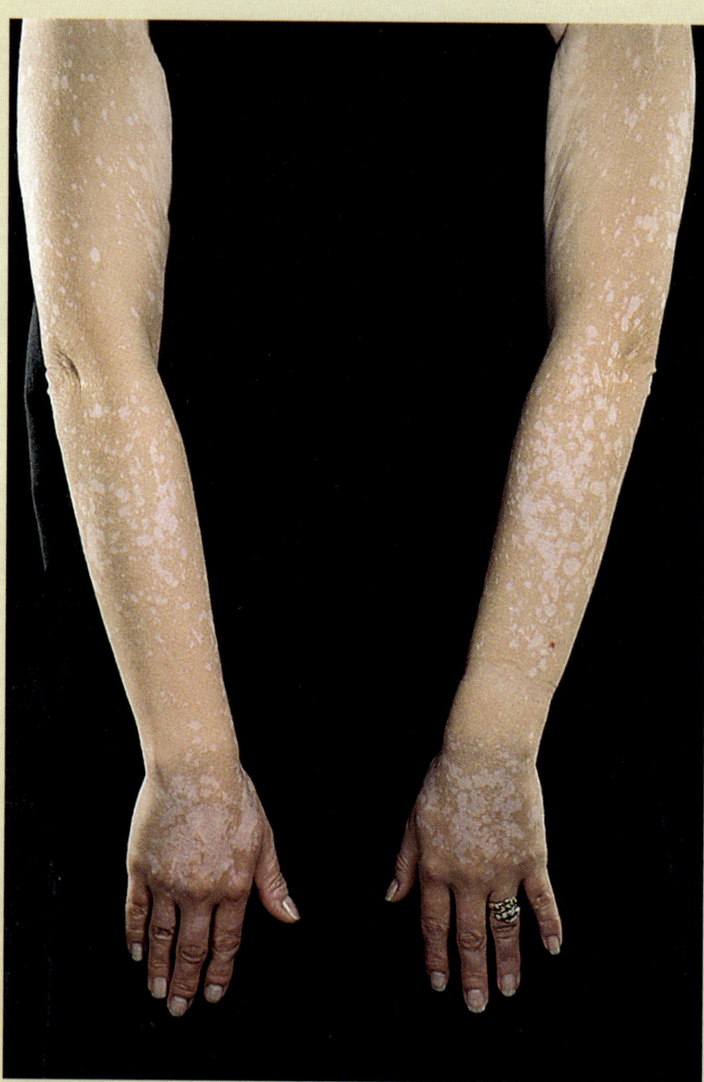

Vitiligo and diabetes mellitus

- Vitiligo is a disorder of skin pigmentation which occurs in approximately 1% of the population and is often familial. It is sometimes associated with diabetes.
- Vitiligo often begins in youth, causing patchy, often symmetrical loss of skin pigmentation at various sites, particularly the face and dorsal aspect of the hands, and sometimes also at the sites of friction and trauma such as on the elbows and knees.
- Vitiligo is thought to result from an auto-immune process, possibly caused by the effect of antibodies against the pigment melanin.
- Vitiligo is classed as one of the organ-specific autoimmune disorders of the thyro-gastric group. This group of disorders also includes pernicious anaemia, Addison's disease, hypoparathyroidism, premature ovarian failure, and Graves' disease, as well as Type 1 diabetes mellitus.
- The histocompatibility antigens commonly associated with this group of disorders are HLA B8, DR3, DR4 and DQ.
- Although many patients with vitiligo may have no other manifestation of autoimmunity, there is a 5–15-fold increase in the incidence of vitiligo in patients with the other thyro-gastric autoimmune disorders.
- The photograph shows the typical appearance of patches of depigmentation on the backs of the hands and arms of a patient with vitiligo associated with Type 1 diabetes.

Palpebral xanthelesmata in diabetes mellitus

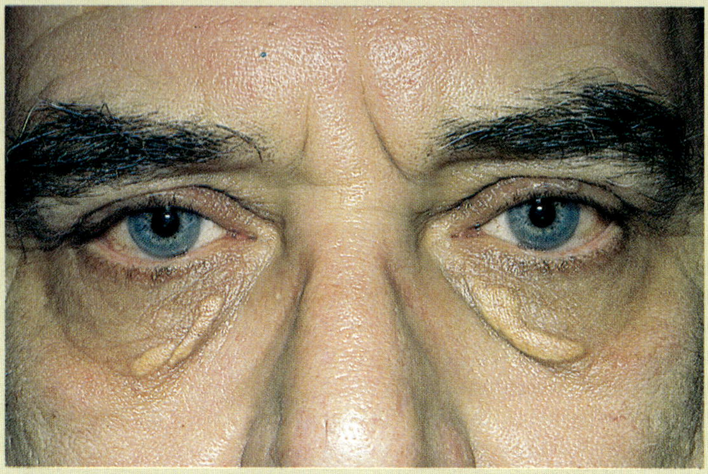

Palpebral xanthelesmata in diabetes mellitus

- Xanthelesmata are raised, yellow plaques on the eyelids, usually near the inner canthus. They are formed by subcutaneous deposition of cholesterol.
- Although xanthelesmata can occur in individuals who have no measurable evidence of dyslipidaemia, their presence is much more likely in people with significant elevations of their plasma total cholesterol levels.
- Xanthelesmata may be found in association with other physical signs of hypercholesterolaemia such as a premature corneal arcus, or the presence of tendon xanthomata in familial hypercholesterolaemic states.
- Hypercholesterolaemia in diabetes may be secondary to associated conditions such as hypothyroidism or nephrotic syndrome, and it is important to exclude these primary conditions, as effective treatment of the underlying cause may reduce the level of plasma cholesterol.
- Hypercholesterolaemia in diabetes constitutes a significant risk factor for accelerated atherosclerotic arterial disease and should be treated actively with appropriate advice about dietary modification and the need for weight reduction and tight glycaemic control as well as management of additional risk factors such as smoking and hypertension. Lipid-lowering drugs should be introduced if cholesterol levels remain elevated.
- The photograph shows typical palpebral xanthelesmata in a man with Type 2 diabetes which had only been diagnosed after he presented with a history of typical angina pectoris. His cholesterol level was significantly elevated but fell to more acceptable levels with appropriate dietary advice, control of his diabetes with an oral hypoglycaemic agent and introduction of cerivastatin. Persuading him to stop smoking proved somewhat more difficult!

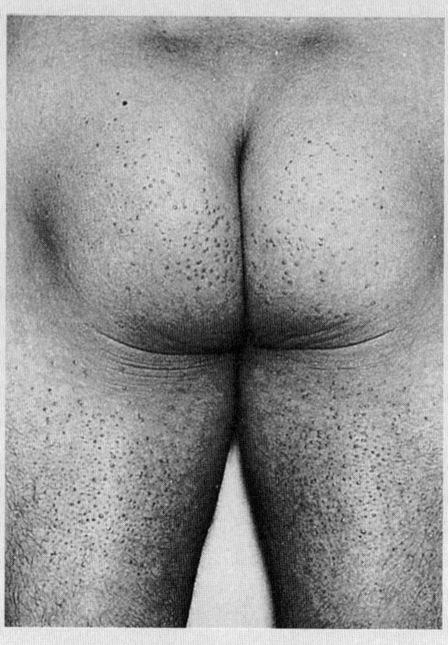

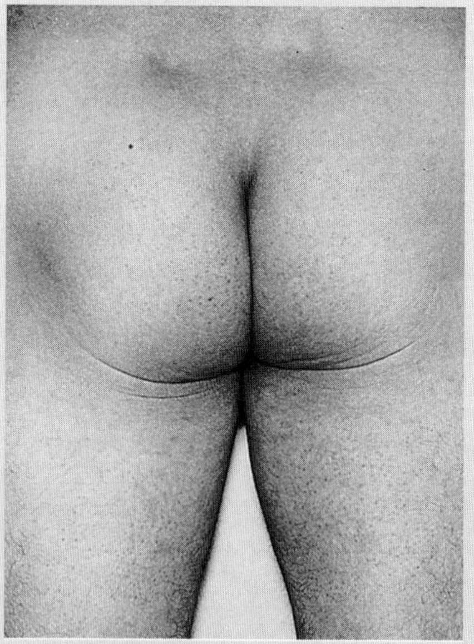

Eruptive xanthomata (xanthoma diabeticorum)

- A small percentage of people whose diabetes is very poorly controlled have greatly raised levels of very low density lipoprotein (VLDL) triglycerides and chylomicrons in the serum. These accumulate not only in macrophages in the liver and spleen but also as collections in the skin. These are known as eruptive xanthomata or xanthoma diabeticorum.
- They occur as small red or yellow nodules up to 5 mm in diameter and are usually located on the buttocks, trunk and on extensor aspects of the extremities.
- The onset is sometimes rapid, and the lesions, which are grouped, usually arise in crops and are sometimes itchy, although itchiness does not often remain a prominent symptom for long.
- The nodules contain mainly triglyceride and a small amount of cholesterol.
- There may be associated lipaemia of the serum which may appear creamy or frankly turbid in the test tube.
- Examination of the optic fundi may reveal the condition of 'lipaemia retinalis' when the blood vessels in the fundi appear milky because of the severe hypertriglyceridaemia.
- The lesions usually regress if lipid levels can be reduced towards normal, usually with improved glycaemic control or with specific lipid-lowering measures.
- The upper photograph shows eruptive xanthomata on the buttocks of a man with poorly controlled diabetes and hypertriglyceridaemia. The lower photograph demonstrates regression of the lesions after appropriate intervention to control the diabetes and lower the triglyceride levels.

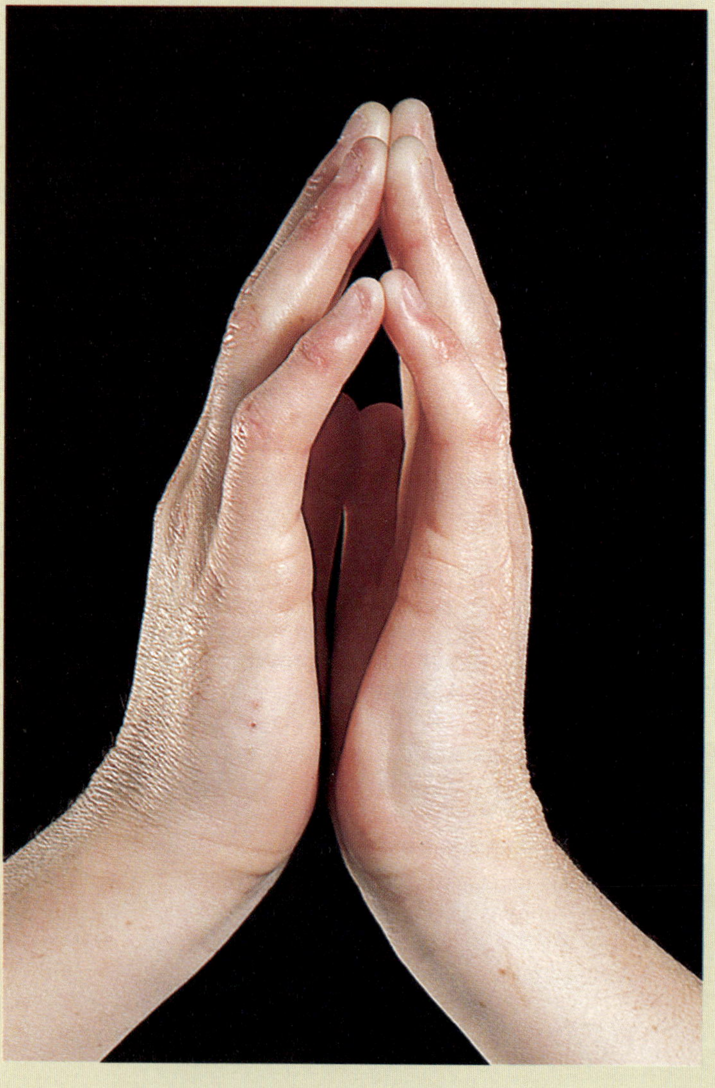

Cheiroarthropathy and limited joint mobility

- People with longstanding diabetes may develop stiffness and limited joint mobility of the fingers with characteristic appearance of tight, shiny, waxy skin over the fingers reminiscent of scleroderma. Typically, this causes an inability to fully extend the fingers at the interphalangeal joints, best demonstrated by asking the patient to place the palms of the hands together ('the prayer sign') or by inability to place the palmar aspect of the hands flat on the surface of a table.
- This condition is known as diabetic cheiroarthropathy, and is commoner than is usually appreciated, occurring in both Type 1 and Type 2 diabetes.
- Diabetic cheiroarthropathy is related to duration and to degree of long-term control of the diabetes, and is said to be associated with the presence of other long-term specific complications of diabetes such as retinopathy. (A common axiom is that 'all patients should pray as they come into the diabetic clinic' . . . and if they demonstrate a positive 'prayer sign' then they should have dilated fundoscopy, foot examination and urine protein estimation.)
- The photograph demonstrates the changes of diabetic cheiroarthropathy, with smooth, shiny skin of the fingers and flexion deformity causing inability to fully extend the fingers giving a positive 'prayer sign'. The patient had been on insulin for Type 1 diabetes since childhood and had developed associated complications in the form of retinopathy, nephropathy and sensorimotor and symptomatic autonomic neuropathy.
- Diabetic cheiroarthropathy may also be associated with stiffness of other joints (elbows, shoulders and knees), with compression neuropathy, especially carpal tunnel syndrome, and with Dupuytren's contracture.
- Frozen shoulder (adhesive capsulitis) is four times commoner in people with diabetes than in the non-diabetic population.

Diabetic miscellany (1)

An astute clinical observer can spot conditions in the diabetic clinic which may adversely affect the prognosis of the diabetes, yet which can be easily overlooked if the emphasis in the clinic is simply on checking the results of tests to monitor blood glucose control and carrying out a standardised screening examination for complications of diabetes, and not on considering diabetes in a wider clinical context.

Inspection of the injection sites in insulin-treated diabetic patients is often only cursorily done, or not done at all by doctors in the busy diabetic clinic setting. Yet, problems with variable insulin absorbtion from injection sites affected by lipohypertrophy or by lipoatrophy may well explain otherwise inexplicable fluctuations in blood glucose levels.

Rarely, diabetes may be associated with infections such as malignant otitis externa which can have severe or even fatal consequences, yet which may present with seemingly trivial symptoms or with signs such as a slight discharge from the external auditory canal. In a busy diabetic clinic setting such innocuous presentations are easily dismissed as being unimportant, but early detection by an alert clinician can lead to early and effective therapy.

Premature loss of bone mass may be a feature of longstanding Type 1 diabetes, leading to diabetic osteopenia or osteoporosis with the possibility of increased risk of subsequent problems such as crush fractures of the vertebrae, or fractures of the hips or long bones.

The availability of methods for the detection of small quantities of albumin in the urine (microalbuminuria) has enabled clinicians to routinely screen in the diabetic clinic for this earliest clinically detectable manifestation of diabetic nephropathy at a stage where therapeutic intervention might retard the otherwise inevitable progress to end-stage renal disease.

Diabetic miscellany (2)

It is easy for a busy clinician to lose sight of the fact that diabetes may occur as a secondary phenomenon in a number of conditions. Examples are acromegaly and Cushing's syndrome. Successful treatment of these primary conditions may lead to the disappearance of diabetes. An astute clinician will always be on the lookout in the diabetic clinic for patients suffering from disorders which might present as secondary diabetes but which require investigation and treatment along different lines from the majority of the other patients attending the clinic.

Dystrophia myotonica is an example of a genetically determined condition in which diabetes is only one part of the phenotype. Such patients may be referred for management of the diabetes, which may be the presenting feature of the underlying inherited disorder. A good clinician will be able to identify the other manifestations of the disorder and offer appropriate advice and genetic counselling to the patient and to family members.

Diabetes is one of many risk factors for cardiovascular disease. Recent awareness of the importance of detecting and treating other risk factors such as lipid abnormalities and hypertension in diabetes, and greater understanding of the possible mechanisms linking these disorders (as elaborated in Professor Reaven's description of the eponymous cardiovascular risk factor syndrome; see Further reading, p. 133) have led to improved therapeutic interventions aimed at reducing overall cardiovascular risk in diabetes. A clinician working in a diabetic clinic therefore has a responsibility not just to concentrate on issues surrounding blood glucose control, but also to undertake an overall cardiovascular risk assessment which should include determining smoking status, lipid levels and blood pressure measurement and recommending dietary or pharmacological intervention to reverse any adverse risk factors identified.

Lipohypertrophy at insulin injection sites

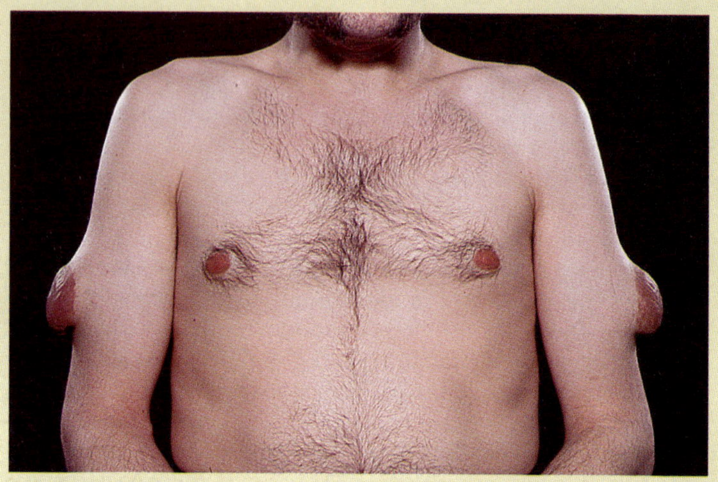

Lipohypertrophy at insulin injection sites

- A local increase in subcutaneous fat can result from repeated injections of insulin into the same site over a period of time. This is relatively common because many people who inject insulin inadvertently fall into the habit of using preferred sites for injection.
- The resulting lipohypertrophy can impair insulin absorbtion from the subcutis and can contribute to erratic glycaemic control.
- Inspection of injection sites is therefore an important part of the examination in the diabetic clinic, with appropriate advice about rotation of injection sites and avoidance of areas of insulin-induced lipohypertrophy.
- The photograph shows an extreme case of a man who had been inserting his twice-daily beef insulin injections into the two preferred sites on his upper arms for 23 years (morning injection: right arm; evening injection: left arm!). As a result, he had developed symmetrical fatty tumours (insulin lipomata) of the upper arms. He was quite happy because his injections were now completely painless and he was unconcerned about the appearance as he never took off his shirt in public!

Lipoatrophy at insulin injection sites

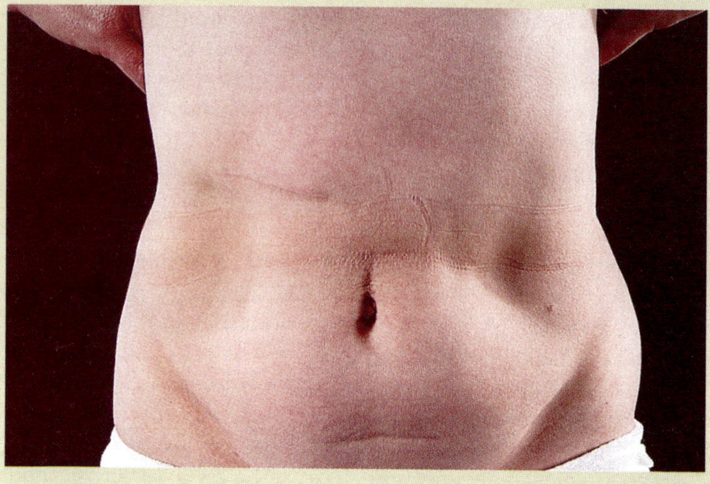

Lipoatrophy at insulin injection sites

- Lipoatrophy is the term used to describe the problem of loss of subcutaneous fat in circumscribed areas at the sites of regular insulin injections, leading to unsightly hollows, as seen in the accompanying photograph of areas of lipoatrophy in a patient who used regularly to inject into the anterior abdomen.
- Sometimes evidence of lipoatrophy can also be found in areas remote from the usual injection sites.
- Lipoatrophy used to be a relatively common complication of subcutaneous insulin injection therapy before highly purified monocomponent animal insulins became widely available.
- Lipoatrophy probably represents a localised immune response to antigenic moieties in the injected insulin.
- Lipoatrophy used to affect up to 25% of patients treated with insulins of animal origin before purifying techniques improved and lessened the immunogenicity of the insulins.
- Human insulin is relatively non-immunogenic, so that problems with lipoatrophy at injection sites are rare (but not unheard of) in patients treated with human insulin.
- In a patient who has developed lipoatrophy after using less pure animal insulin, resolution of the lesions can occur after a change to a more highly purified insulin. The patient should be advised to inject the new insulin into the skin around the edges of the areas of lipoatrophy as this is said to speed the filling in of the hollows.
- The photograph shows extensive areas of lipoatrophy at the injection sites on the abdomen in a patient who had been using beef insulin for some years.

Malignant otitis externa (and other severe infections of the head and neck)

- This rare condition is an infection of the external ear which usually occurs in people with diabetes and which can have very serious consequences. The word 'malignant' refers to the serious nature of the condition rather than to any histological evidence of malignancy in the generally accepted sense.
- Elderly people with diabetes are particularly prone to this serious infection, which has only rarely been recorded in non-diabetic people.
- The infecting organism is usually *Pseudomonas aeruginosa*.
- The patient presents with otalgia, otorrhoea and poor control of the diabetes.
- Necrotic granulation tissue from which the Pseudomonas may be cultured, is found in the external auditory meatus.
- The infection spreads to involve the temporal bone. Infected granulation tissue can also erode deeply into the middle and inner ear and the bone of the skull base.
- Extension into the brain may occur, with involvement of the roots and nuclei of the lower cranial nerves causing multiple cranial nerve palsies and brain-stem syndromes. The great vessels of the neck may be involved and the condition may lead to serious neurological morbidity and may even prove fatal.
- Treatment with anti-pseudomonal antibiotics, usually given parenterally, combined in some cases with surgical drainage and clearance of infected material, may stop the progress of the disease.
- People with diabetes also exhibit particular susceptibility to two other severe infections of the head and neck, namely rhinocerebral mucormycosis (an extensive, life-threatening fungal infection beginning in the nasal passages and sinuses and often extending into the orbit and the cerebrum) and endophthalmitis (a severe infection of the vitreal contents of the eye which may occur post-operatively or be secondary to trauma or to bacteraemia).

Osteoporosis in diabetes mellitus (diabetic osteopenia)

- Bone mineral density has been shown to be reduced in some patients with Type 1, insulin-dependent diabetes. This has been referred to as 'diabetic osteopenia'.
- By contrast, bone mineral density has been demonstrated to be normal or even increased in patients with Type 2, non-insulin-dependent diabetes.
- The pathogenesis of diabetic osteopenia is not completely understood, but is considered to be multifactorial, possibly involving lack of growth factors, abnormalities of vitamin D metabolism and disturbances of parathyroid hormone production and action.
- Abnormalities of parathyroid hormone and vitamin D metabolism are likely to be of particular relevance when diabetic osteopenia occurs in patients with established diabetic renal disease.
- Diabetic osteopenia may be found in association with other long-term complications of diabetes in patients with Type 1 diabetes.
- Patients with longstanding diabetes who have elevated urinary albumin excretion rates (positive microalbuminuria) but otherwise normal kidney function have been shown to have significantly lower bone mineral density than patients with diabetes of similar type and duration who have normal kidney function with normal urinary albumin excretion rates (negative microalbuminuria).
- The clinical significance of diabetic osteopenia is not clear. Some studies have shown increased fracture rates in patients with Type 1, insulin-dependent diabetes, whilst other studies have not shown an increase in fracture rates in such patients.

Disorders associated with secondary diabetes: Cushing's syndrome

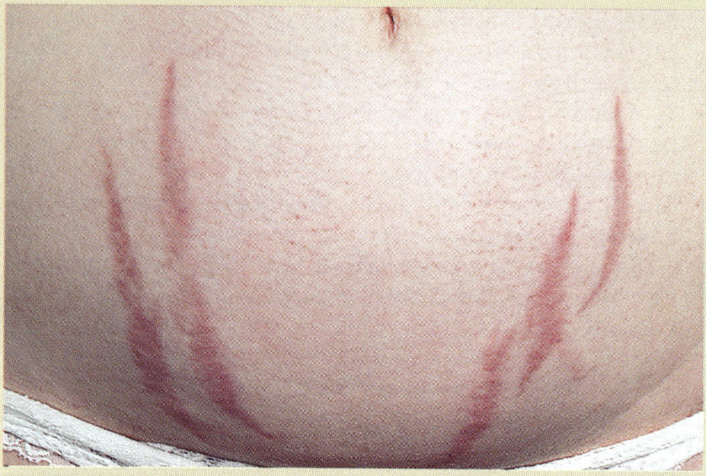

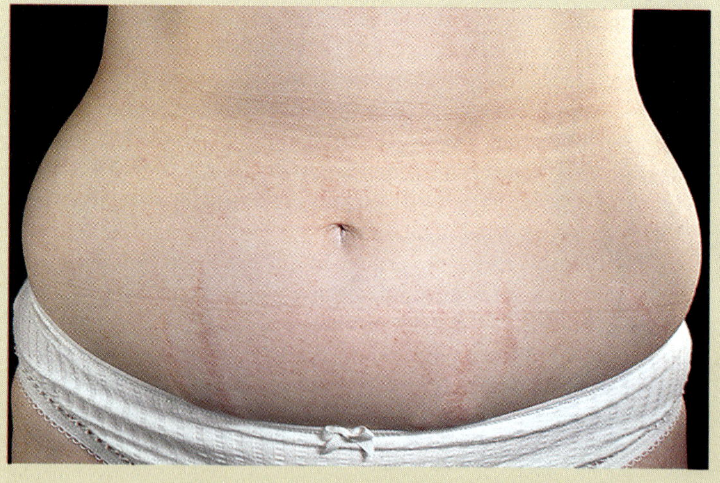

Disorders associated with secondary diabetes: Cushing's syndrome

- Cortisol and other glucocorticoids increase hepatic gluconeogenesis and impair the peripheral tissue utilisation of glucose, thus causing a tendency to hyperglycaemia.
- About 30% of patients with Cushing's syndrome will have a high blood glucose level. Exogenous steroid drugs can have the same effect, especially when used in high doses. Patients on steroid therapy should therefore be monitored regularly for glycosuria and hyperglycaemia.
- This photograph is of the abdomen of a female patient who was referred to the diabetic clinic by her family practitioner because of hypertension and glycosuria associated with increasing obesity. Diabetes was confirmed on blood glucose testing. She had put on a significant amount of weight in a relatively short period of time and had noticed weakness and possible wasting of her limb muscles, particularly those of the thighs. It was only after an astute medical student had drawn attention to the active abdominal striae that it dawned upon her medical attendants that they were not dealing with just another difficult woman with obesity-related diabetes and hypertension, but that she was also exhibiting other typical features of hypercortisolism (Cushing's syndrome): a plethoric 'moon face'; 'buffalo hump' or interscapular fat pad; truncal obesity with striae; bruising; and evidence of a proximal myopathy. Endocrinological investigations confirmed the diagnosis of cortisol excess and an adrenal mass was demonstrated on abdominal computerised tomography (CT) scanning. She was referred to a surgeon and underwent surgical removal of an adrenal adenoma after pre-operative metyrapone therapy to suppress the steroid excess. She made an uneventful recovery with successful amelioration of both the hypertension and diabetes, and regression of the abdominal striae, as shown in the second photograph which was taken some weeks post-operatively.

Disorders associated with secondary diabetes: acromegaly

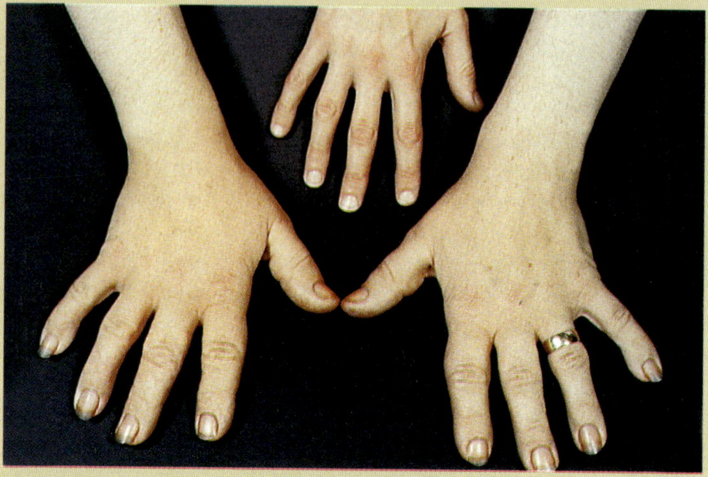

Disorders associated with secondary diabetes: acromegaly

- Growth hormone stimulates lipolysis causing peripheral mobilisation of glycerol and therefore antagonising the peripheral effects of insulin.
- Approximately 25% of patients with acromegaly will develop diabetes, especially those who have a family history of diabetes. Cure of the acromegaly after successful pituitary adenomectomy or hypophysectomy can result in a dramatic increase in insulin sensitivity leading to significant improvement or even cure of the diabetes.
- It has been suggested that growth hormone may have a role in the pathogenesis of proliferative diabetic retinopathy, possibly acting through intermediary growth factors in the retina. Hypophysectomy used to be employed as an often successful treatment of advanced diabetic retinal disease.
- The photograph is of the hands of a patient with acromegaly, with the hand of the clinic nurse for comparison—demonstrating the gross enlargement of the extremities which raised the suspicion of acromegaly as a cause of the hyperglycaemia which had been the reason for the patient's referral to hospital. She had severe diabetes, with one episode at least of life-threatening ketoacidosis. She was treated with twice-daily insulin injections, and went on to develop proliferative diabetic retinopathy requiring laser therapy. However, after trans-sphenoidal pituitary adenomectomy followed by radiotherapy, cure of the acromegaly was achieved with growth hormone levels persistently less than 10 mU/l, and suppressing completely with a 50-g oral glucose load. Normoglycaemia was achieved on a sugar-free diet alone, and the retinopathy showed signs of marked regression.

Disorders associated with secondary diabetes: dystrophia myotonica

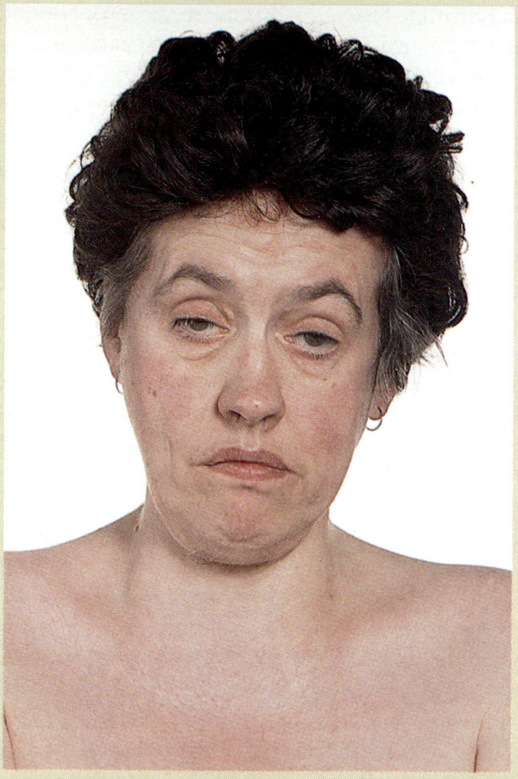

Disorders associated with secondary diabetes: dystrophia myotonica

- Diabetes is often found in this form of muscular dystrophy which is characterised by myotonia with muscular weakness and wasting, particularly of the masseters, temporalis and sternocleidomastoid muscles, with ptosis giving a distinctive facial appearance.
- Other features include frontal baldness, cataract, gonadal atrophy, cardiomyopathy, pulmonary ventilatory impairment, oesophageal smooth muscle involvement and mild intellectual impairment.
- The diabetes probably results from insulin resistance and responds better to insulin therapy than to oral hypoglycaemic agents.
- The condition results from autosomal dominant inheritance of a genetic mutation on chromosome 19 which causes an unstable DNA sequence known as a trinucleotide repeat expansion. This interferes with normal function of the protein kinase gene and adjacent genes.
- Each generation shows progressively worse manifestations of the disorder at an earlier onset. This is because of the genetic phenomenon known as 'anticipation', because the size of the trinucleotide gene expansion on the chromosome increases with each successive generation, disrupting more and more of the normal gene function.
- The photograph is of a patient who was referred to the diabetic clinic from the orthopaedic ward following admission with a fractured neck of femur. There was glycosuria, and diabetes was confirmed on blood testing. The patient was wearing a wig to conceal frontal baldness and had myopathic facies with bilateral ptosis, wasted sternocleidomastoid muscles and palatal speech. The grip was weak, with obvious myotonia. There were bilateral cataracts. There was a history of cataract in several paternal family members and an uncle had died in middle age of a muscle disorder. Electromyography (EMG) gave the pathognomonic 'dive bomber' sign of myotonia when the audio channel was turned up. The diabetes responded to treatment with twice-daily insulin injections. The patient and her immediate family were referred for genetic counselling.

Microalbuminuria

- The term 'microalbuminuria' is used to describe elevation of the urinary albumin excretion rate below the proteinuric ('dipstick-positive') level.
- Microalbuminuria is present when there is an increase in the urinary albumin excretion rate to between 30 and 300 mg in 24 hours. For the diagnosis to be confirmed this must be detected in at least two out of three consecutive, clean, timed urine samples.
- Albumin/creatinine ratio on early morning urine samples is the single most sensitive screening test, but testing of random urine samples offers greater convenience at the expense of reduced sensitivity. A finding on screening of an increase in the albumin/creatinine ratio to more than 2.5 mg/mmol in men, or more than 3.5 mg/mmol in women, should be followed by repeat testing of an early morning urine sample. If the abnormality persists on repeat testing then formal quantitative testing of timed samples is indicated.
- Microalbuminuria is the earliest clinically detectable manifestation of diabetic nephropathy and predates the development of end-stage renal disease in patients with Type 1 and Type 2 diabetes.
- Microalbuminuria also predicts excess cardiovascular risk in Type 2 diabetes, with a positive test predicting a two-fold excess mortality over the next 8 years and therefore identifying a subset of patients who may benefit from aggressive treatment of cardiovascular disease risk factors.
- Treating patients with microalbuminuria with angiotensin converting enzyme (ACE) inhibitors slows the progression to overt proteinuria in Type 1 and Type 2 diabetes, even in patients who do not have hypertension.
- The results of the DCCT in 1993 demonstrated that maintenance of excellent glycaemic control by intensive insulin therapy in patients with Type 1 diabetes can prevent the development of microalbuminuria (primary prevention), or retard its progression when already established (secondary prevention).

Hypertension and its treatment in diabetes

- Hypertension may exist in association with glucose intolerance or frank diabetes as part of the syndrome which results from insulin resistance and consequent hyperinsulinaemia. It may also be secondary to renal damage in both Type 1 and Type 2 diabetes. Hypertension may also result from primary conditions such as Cushing's syndrome or acromegaly which may be associated with secondary diabetes.
- The management of hypertension may therefore be different in patients with diabetes of different aetiologies.
- Management may also differ depending on the presence or absence of vascular or other complications of the diabetes.
- Effective control of blood pressure slows down the decline in renal function in established diabetic nephropathy.
- Extrapolation from the results of trials in people without diabetes suggests the possibility of benefit from antihypertensive treatment in prevention of cardiovascular and cerebrovascular disease in diabetic people with associated hypertension.
- Beta-blockers are relatively contraindicated in people with diabetes treated with insulin or with sulphonylurea drugs because they might mask the adrenergic symptoms of hypoglycaemia and may have an adverse effect on the normal counter-regulatory response to hypoglycaemia. Hypoglycaemia might therefore come on without warning and might be more profound and more prolonged. Beta-blockers might also be contraindicated in people with diabetes and arterial insufficiency as they may increase the risks of peripheral ischaemia.
- Thiazide diuretics are not ideal antihypertensive agents for people with diabetes as they might worsen glycaemic control as well as precipitating hyperuricaemia.
- ACE inhibitors have been shown to reverse microalbuminuria.
- Calcium-channel blockers may also have a potentially beneficial effect in reversing microalbuminuria.
- Alpha-blockers may alter adverse lipid profiles in a potentially beneficial direction.
- Antihypertensive agents may worsen the effects of diabetic autonomic neuropathy, especially postural hypotension and erectile impotence.

Lipids in diabetes

- There is a three-fold increase in risk of coronary heart disease in patients with Type 1 diabetes, and a six-fold increase in risk in patients with Type 2 diabetes, independent of the other major risk factors.
- Lipid and lipoprotein abnormalities are common in diabetes, and probably contribute to the increased cardiovascular risk.
- The commonest lipid abnormalities in uncontrolled diabetes are hypertriglyceridaemia with an excess of VLDL, and elevation of total cholesterol with reduced levels of the potentially protective high density lipoprotein (HDL) cholesterol.
- Cholesterol levels may also be elevated as a secondary phenomenon in diabetic patients with nephropathy and nephrotic syndrome. Patients with diabetic ketoacidosis may have a severe elevation of blood lipids resulting in frankly lipaemic blood plasma. These lipid abnormalities can be corrected by reversing the underlying metabolic defect.
- Initial treatment of lipid abnormalities in diabetes is to optimise glucose control with appropriate dietary modification and oral hypoglycaemic drugs or insulin. Advice should include instruction about a low-saturated fat, low-cholesterol diet and reduction of body weight, as well as about other lifestyle modifications such as smoking cessation and increased exercise to further decrease cardiovascular risk.
- If lipid levels remain altered in a potentially adverse direction despite the above measures, then lipid-lowering drugs should be introduced.
- Hypertriglyceridaemia and mixed hyperlipidaemia respond well to fibrate drugs some of which (such as bezafibrate) can also have a beneficial effect on glucose levels.
- Elevated total cholesterol levels usually respond to the use of a statin such as simvastatin or pravastatin. These drugs usually have no effect on triglyceride levels although some of the newer statins such as atorvastatin or cerivastatin can lower triglyceride levels as well as affecting cholesterol synthesis.

Insulin resistance and the metabolic syndrome

- The insulin molecule interacts with insulin receptors located in the plasma membrane. This initiates a cascade of reactions at post-receptor level, which control the enzyme steps regulating glucose, fatty acid and amino acid metabolism.
- Defects at receptor or post-receptor level may reduce the action of insulin, resulting in diminished sensitivity of peripheral tissues to its effects. Insulin resistance of this sort appears to be partly an inherited characteristic and partly related to physiological variables including increased abdominal adiposity as expressed by the 'waist/hip ratio' in men.
- In response to insulin resistance, the beta cells of the islets of Langerhans are stimulated to produce greater amounts of insulin, leading to a state of basal hyperinsulinaemia.
- Prolonged hyperinsulinaemia can lead to systemic arterial hypertension.
- Hyperinsulinaemia can lead to increased VLDL and LDL and decreased HDL cholesterol levels, as well as hypertriglyceridaemia.
- Hyperinsulinaemia is also associated with other abnormalities including high fibrinogen levels.
- Prolonged beta-cell hyperfunction resulting from the need to overcome tissue insulin resistance ultimately leads to beta-cell fatigue. This results initially in a state of impaired glucose tolerance, and finally in beta-cell failure with inadequate basal and post-prandial insulin levels giving rise to frank diabetes.
- In some people, therefore, the onset of clinically obvious diabetes is the end result of a process which may have been ongoing for a considerable time. The state of diabetes is only one manifestation of the whole syndrome which results from the state of peripheral insulin resistance and which is characterised by a collection of a number of cardiovascular risk factors including hyperinsulinaemia, hypertension, hypertriglyceridaemia, low HDL cholesterol, high fibrinogen levels and hyperglycaemia.
- This may explain why a number of people with Type 2 diabetes already have established vascular disease at presentation.

Diabetic clinic records

Accurate recording of clinical information in a form which is easily accessible is essential. Currently, the majority of hospital clinics rely on handwritten paper records stored in the patients' case notes. The standard of note keeping can sometimes be poor. Even in the best organised diabetic clinic it is not always possible for the same doctor to see the patient at each clinic visit—there are hospital doctors in training, research fellows and other career grade physicians working in the diabetic clinic. Nurses, dietitians, chiropodists and other health professionals should also have access to medical notes and their own notes should form an integral part of the patient record. Well kept and readable clinic records can ensure that information about a patient's diabetes is immediately available to all the members of the multidisciplinary team who are involved in helping and advising the patient about the management of the diabetes.

Examples are given in the following section of clinic record sheets, annual review sheets, and diabetic liaison nursing, dietitian and chiropody request forms which are currently in use in our diabetic clinics in Doncaster. These may be far from perfect but they represent an attempt to standardise information collection in the case notes in a reasonably structured way.

Manually created paper casenotes look likely to be replaced by computerised patient records, providing accurate data storage and retrieval with facilities for rapid electronic communication. It will be important for all health districts to develop a strategy for using information technology to improve the delivery of clinical care to people with diabetes, but it is vital that this should be achieved without compromising patient confidentiality or safety.

Organisation of diabetes care

Responsibility for the care of a chronic condition such as diabetes rests with many different people. The primary care physician provides continuity of medical advice for the majority of patients, some of whom may never need to be referred to the hospital service. Other patients with diabetes who are difficult to treat, or who are pregnant, or have advanced diabetic complications or other illness, may require almost exclusively hospital specialist-based care.

Most diabetic people should receive most of their care in the primary care setting but with occasional hospital specialist review. Jointly agreed guidelines on shared care can greatly facilitate this arrangement, ensuring reasonable uniformity of treatment goals and modalities. It is important that such guidelines should be formally revised at regular intervals in order to take into account changes which can happen in a rapidly developing field of medicine.

Diabetes specialist nurses can liaise between hospital and primary care and can provide valuable support and education for patients and their carers in coming to terms with a condition whose diagnosis has far-reaching consequences and which requires active monitoring and management on a day-to-day basis.

Diet is the mainstay of treatment of all types of diabetes and the professional dietitian has an extremely important part to play in advising and educating patients about the intricacies of healthy eating.

The chiropodist is another vital member of the diabetes team, providing treatment and education to reduce the significant burden of morbidity associated with diabetic foot problems.

The organisation of diabetes care involving so many disparate groups can be complex. The establishment of local diabetes service advisory groups can play a key role in ensuring appropriate and efficient use of available health resources for the good of the population of people with diabetes.

DIABETES FOLLOW-UP RECORD	*AFFIX LABEL HERE IF AVAILABLE* Unit Number: 123456 Surname: AHOLIC Forename(s): CHOC

Year of Onset: 1993 Age at Onset: 39 Insulin Started: 1995

Cataract 1993 ☒ Retinopathy ☐ Poor vision ☐ Nephropathy ☐
Peripheral Neuropathy ☐ Autonomic Neuropathy ☐ Amyotrophy ☐ Foot Problems ☐
Peripheral Vascular Disease ☐ Ischaemic Heart Disease ☐ Hypertension ☐ Cerebrovascular Disease ☐
Other Problems: Duodenal ulcer 1987
Height: ......(cm) Ideal Body Weight: ......(kg) Smoker? Yes / (No) Stopped 1989

Date: 27/12/94 Weight: 78kg	Urine Protein	Urine Ketone	Urine Glucose	Blood Glucose	HbA_{1-c}	Home (Urine) / Blood Tests: B/fast	Lunch	Tea
	0	0	++	16.4	8.8%	1/4% - 1/2%	⟶	1% - 2%

Comments:	B.P.	Full check done?	Treatment:
Feeling tired. Some nocturia Start Metformin Refer to Diabetic liaison	140/80	(Yes)/~~No~~ Next Appt. (2/12)	a.m. Diet alone p.m. Diet: Sugar free, low fat

Date: 10/2/95 Weight: 75kg	Urine Protein	Urine Ketone	Urine Glucose	Blood Glucose	HbA_{1-c}	Home (Urine) / Blood Tests: B/fast	Lunch	Tea
	0	0	0	8.2	/	0 - 1/10%		1/10% - 1/2%

Comments:	B.P.	Full check done?	Treatment:
Metformin not tolerated because of bowel upset ∴ G.P. started Tolbutamide - feels better No osmotic symptoms	130/80	~~Yes~~/(No) Next Appt. (6/12)	a.m. T 500 mg p.m. T 500 mg Diet: ⟶ Dietitian for review

Date: 16/8/95 Weight: 74kg	Urine Protein	Urine Ketone	Urine Glucose	Blood Glucose	HbA_{1-c}	Home (Urine) / ~~Blood~~ Tests: B/fast	Lunch	Tea
	0	0	+++	17.2	8.4%	1%	⟶	1% - 2%

Comments:	B.P.	Full check done?	Treatment:
Poor control despite increasing Tolbutamide to 1g T.D.S. ⟶ symptomatic. Refer to Diabetic Liaison Sister to learn Home Blood testing. MAY NEED INSULIN.	130/75	~~Yes~~/(No) Next Appt. (2/12)	a.m. T 1g T 1g p.m. T 1g Diet: Says he's sticking to a strict diet.

Date: 24/10/95 Weight: 80kg	Urine Protein	Urine Ketone	Urine Glucose	Blood Glucose	HbA_{1-c}	Home Urine / (Blood) Tests: B/fast	Lunch	Tea
	(+)	0	0	9.2	7.1%	7-9	9 - 11(- 17)	4 - 7.9

Comments:	B.P.	Full check done?	Treatment:
Check MSU Diabetic Liaison Sister has started him on insulin. No problems. Feels "great". One mild hypo. Injects ✓ Do full check next time.	130/80	~~Yes~~/(No) Next Appt. (3/12)	HUMULIN M-3 a.m. (28) p.m. (12) Diet: Review spaced CHO diet.

T=Tolbutamide C=Chlorpropamide G=Glibenclamide GZ=Gliclazide M=Metformin A=Acarbose

The diabetic clinic follow-up record

- Patient details are at the top of the sheet, as well as the date of onset of diabetes; the patient's age at onset; and if on insulin, the date that insulin was started. Other details include indications of known complications; associated hypertension; ischaemic heart disease; history; height; and ideal body weight. This section is updated as and when necessary.
- The form contains enough space for several clinic entries so that a cumulative record can be built up over several visits.
- An entry is made every time the patient attends the diabetic clinic.
- The following information is collected and entered before the patient comes in to see the doctor: date; weight; urine dipstick test for protein, ketones and glucose; blood glucose level; HbA_{1-c} (either measured 'on line' in the clinic, or by arrangement with the laboratory a week beforehand); and blood pressure.
- The clinic doctor enters details of the present treatment for diabetes, indicating doses and timing; the home urine or blood glucose test profiles; and dietary details. Also, a comment is entered in the relevant section giving details of any problems, changes in treatment or other relevant clinical information. If a full check is done, this is recorded (and details of the full check are entered on a separate diabetic full check sheet). Arrangements for the next clinic appointment are recorded.

The fictitious example record is of a Mr Choc Aholic whose diabetes was diagnosed at age 39 in 1993 when his astute family practitioner detected glycosuria on routine urine testing before referring him to the ophthalmologist for an opinion about a developing cataract. Random blood sugar at presentation was 16 mmol/l, and Mr Aholic admitted to fairly recent onset of symptoms of tiredness, thirst and urinary frequency. He was started on a sugar-free diet, taught how to carry out home urine tests and referred to the Type 2 education sessions run in the local hospital diabetic centre by the diabetic liaison nurses and the dietitians. At first, his diabetes was fairly well controlled, and he was initially followed up in the practice diabetic clinic.

- He was referred for assessment in the hospital diabetic clinic at the end of 1994 because urine tests showed persistent glycosuria and his symptoms had returned. He was started on metformin, and a full diabetic check was carried out at that presenting visit.
- Metformin was not tolerated so the family practitioner started treatment with tolbutamide. At the next hospital clinic visit he was sent to the dietitian for review, and things appeared to be settling. However, over succeeding months control deteriorated and tolbutamide was increased to its maximum dose.
- In August 1995 the diabetic liaison nurses were asked to teach him how to carry out home capillary blood glucose testing and to monitor him at home, and start insulin if persistent poor control was observed despite strict compliance with diet. He was subsequently started on twice-daily fixed mixture insulin.
- At the most recent visit in October 1995, persistent proteinuria was noted and mid-stream urine was checked. It was noted that a full check would need to be done at the next visit.

DIABETIC CLINIC CHECK	
	UNIT No. 123456
	SURNAME AHOLIC
	FIRST NAMES CHOC

CHECK CARRIED OUT BY DR.: JONES

DATE 2 8 0 1 9 6

URINE – ALBUMIN	++
URINE – GLUCOSE	+
WEIGHT	84•0
PULSE (/MIN.)	78
REGULAR (O). IRREGULAR (I)	0
BLOOD PRESSURE	140 / 80
BLOOD GLUCOSE	12•8

SMOKER 0

CIGS/DAY 0

EYES VISUAL ACUITY

Worse than 6/60 = 6/99
Blind = 6/00

		R. EYE	L. EYE
UNCORRECTED =	0.	6/ 24	6/ 36
SPECTACLES =	1.	6/ 12	6/ 18
PINHOLE =	2.	6/ 12	6/ 18

if 0 or 1 worse than 6/12

enter code for best result 1

CATARACT nil = 0 mild = 1 retina not clearly seen = 9	1	1

FUNDI (pupils dilated)

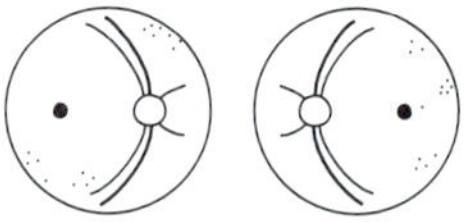

R L

Blots and dots

	R	L
background retinopathy	1	1
proliferative retinopathy	0	0
vitreous haemorrhage	0	0
retinitis proliferans	0	0

nil = 0, present = 1, retina not visible = 9

NO = 0
YES = 1

attending ophthalmologist	1
referred to ophthalmologist	0

INVESTIGATIONS TICK - ALWAYS DO MSU, u&e and GHB	
FBC and ESR	
GHB	✓
MSU	✓
u & e	✓
24hr URINE PROTEIN	✓
IVP	
CXR	
ECG	
LFT'S	
B12 and FOLATE	
other:	

LIMBS

	R	L
FEMORAL	1	1
POPLITEAL	1	1
D. PEDIS	0	0
POST TIBIAL	1	1
KNEE REFLEX	1	1
ANKLE REFLEX	0	0
FEET – LIGHT TOUCH (Diminished=0)	1	1
FEET – VIBRATION (Diminished=0)	0	0
FOOT ULCER	0	0
ATTENDING CHIROPODIST	0	
REFERRED TO CHIROPODIST	1	

CODES
ABSENT/NO=0
PRESENT/YES=1
AMPUTATION=9

MEDICATION:

HUMULIN M-3
28 units morning
12 units evening

Morning insulin to be increased to 30 units.

OTHER PROBLEMS

ISCHAEMIC HEART DISEASE	0
CEREBROVASCULAR DISEASE	0
NEPHROPATHY	?
PYELONEPHRITIS	0
AUTONOMIC NEUROPATHY	0
PAST/PRESENT HYPERTHYROIDISM	0
PAST/PRESENT HYPOTHYROIDISM	0
PERNICIOUS ANAEMIA	0

1. DUODENAL ULCER 1987
2.
3.

INJECTION SITES:

Thighs slightly lumpy
Abdomen O.K.

COMMENTS: Advised about further insulin dose adjustment and avoidance of preferred injection sites on thighs.

CHANGE RECALL INTERVAL TO ☐ MONTHS HBA_{1-c} ☐ %   PLASMA CREATININE ☐ mmol/l

The diabetic clinic check record (annual review sheet)

- At the top of the form are patient details, the date of the examination and the identity of the doctor who carried it out.
- The clinic nurse records: urine dipstick test for albumin and glucose; patient's weight; number of cigarettes smoked; pulse rate and regularity; blood pressure; and blood glucose level.
- Visual acuity is tested, corrected for refractive error with the patient's own glasses if appropriate. If the visual acuity does not correct to better than 6/12, or if the patient has not brought glasses, further correction for refractive error is attempted with a pinhole. Tropicamide 0.5% or 1% drops are then instilled (unless there is a contraindication).
- The doctor undertakes dilated fundoscopy, indicating the presence (1) or absence (0) of cataract; background retinopathy; proliferative retinopathy; vitreous haemorrhage; and retinitis proliferans. Inability to see the fundus clearly is indicated when appropriate (9). The doctor records if the patient is already attending or is to be referred to the ophthalmologist.
- The doctor records the presence (1) or absence (0) of femoral, popliteal, posterior tibial, dorsalis pedis pulses; knee and ankle reflexes; and light touch and vibration sensation at the feet. If an amputation has been carried out, this can be indicated (9). The presence (1) or absence (0) of a foot ulcer can be recorded, and an indication can be given of attendance at or referral to the chiropodist.
- The patient's treatment, and any changes in the treatment, can be recorded, and the presence of injection site problems recorded. The presence (1) or absence (0) of ischaemic heart disease; cerebrovascular disease; autonomic neuropathy; thyroid dysfunction; pernicious anaemia, and any other relevant conditions can be recorded.
- Details of investigations to be carried out are indicated, and there is room for a comment at the end.

The fictitious example is of a diabetic clinic check carried out on Mr Choc Aholic by Dr Jones on the 28 January 1996.

- He was weighed by the clinic nurse at 84 kg. Urine tests showed proteinuria and glycosuria and his pulse was measured at a regular 78 beats/minute with a blood pressure of 140/80. His capillary blood glucose value was 12.8 mmol/l and he was recorded as being a non-smoker.
- Visual acuity, uncorrected, was 6/24 in the right eye and 6/36 in the left eye, correcting with glasses to 6/12 and 6/18, respectively, with no improvement when a pinhole was used.
- There was a mild cataract seen on examination of both eyes, but the optic fundi were visible and showed evidence of background retinopathy with 'blot' haemorrhages and 'dot' microaneurysms. The patient was already being followed up in the ophthalmological clinic.
- All pulses were present, with the exception of the dorsalis pedis pulses which were diminished bilaterally. There was diminution of the ankle jerks bilaterally although the knee jerks were preserved.
- Light touch sensation was preserved in both feet but vibration sense was diminished. There was no foot ulcer, but the patient was referred to the chiropodist.
- Treatment was recorded and changes noted. Routine blood and urine tests were requested as well as a 24-hour urinary protein excretion estimation. Injection sites were inspected and advice was given on avoiding preferred sites.

DIABETIC LIAISON SISTER'S REFERRAL

Name of Patient: CHOC AHOLIC Address: 2, SUGAR LUMPS SWEETOOTH Age: 40	Date: 27th December 1994 ~~Urgent~~ (Non-urgent)
G.P. DR. JECKYLL	District Nursing Sister Sister B. M. Strip

Current Treatment:

Sugar free, low fat diet alone until now.
- I am starting him on METFORMIN 500 mg B.D. today.

Reason for Referral:

Diabetes diagnosed 1993.

Has been on diet alone since then, but now has persistent glycosuria and osmotic symptoms.

Please review dietary compliance and check self-monitoring technique, and give general information and advice.

Date and Method of Notification (e.g. 'Phone)

Telephone No. 654321
(works number - between 8 am & 3 pm.)

Referred by: Emyr Jones (DR. JONES)

Diabetic liaison service referral form

- In some countries a specialist diabetic liaison nursing service has been established, providing an invaluable resource linking hospital specialist, primary care team and the patients and their families. The diabetes nurses are available to provide information about diabetes and its treatment, to educate patients in practical as well as therapeutic aspects of diabetes care and home monitoring, to supervise and advise on changes in therapy and to provide support and access to specialist advice.
- The diabetic liaison service is available to patients, to family practitioners and the practice-based nurses, and to the hospital-based specialists and their teams. There is often a big demand for their services.
- It is therefore vitally important that requests for their involvement in patient management are clearly written, and that full details are given as indicated on the form of patient details, including full address and name of family practitioner, district nurse (if known), current treatment, and especially of the reason for referral. An indication of the degree of urgency of the request is important, and clear instructions of the best time and method to communicate with the patient (e.g. daytime telephone number, etc.).

DIET REQUEST SHEET	*AFFIX LABEL HERE IF AVAILABLE* Unit Number............123456............ Surname............AHOLIC............ Forename(s)............CHOC............

THIS SECTION TO BE COMPLETED BY DOCTOR/NURSE

D.o.B.:.23.03.54.......... Male/Female   Consultant/G.P.:..E.W.J...........

Clinical/Details/Diagnosis:
Type II Diabetes - on diet alone since diagnosis in 1993. Control poor - starting Metformin.

Ward/Clinic:.........Diabetic Clinic..........
Diet or Service Required: Please review sugar free, low fat, high fibre diet
Signature:..EW Jones..........

(THIS SECTION TO BE COMPLETED BY DIETITIAN (ONLY RELEVANT DETAILS REQUIRED))

Diet Sheet:

Daily Allowances:

Bread..........................portions   Protein..........................g/day
Milk..........................pint(s)   Carbohydrate..........................g/day
Fat..........................oz   Distribution • • • • • •
Fruit..........................portions   Supplements........................./day

DIET HISTORY:

Breakfast:

Mid-morning:

Mid-day:

Mid-afternoon:

Evening Meal:

Supper:

CHECK-LIST:

Meat/Fish/Egg..........................
Bread/Cereal..........................
Fats..........................
Milk/Cheese..........................
Sugar..........................
Fruit..........................
Vegetables/Salad..........................
Snacks..........................
Confectionery..........................
Beverages..........................
Alcohol..........................
Take-away meals..........................
Supplements..........................
Cooking Methods (state)..........................
Other (state)..........................

Social History /Exercise:..........................

Diet request card and record

- Diet is the mainstay of treatment for both Type 1 and Type 2 diabetes. The current attitude is to advise a high-fibre, high-carbohydrate, low-fat diet, with calorie restriction for the overweight patient.
- There are several principles which are applicable to all patients with diabetes.
  - Simple sugar avoidance is the first and simplest line of dietary management.
  - A diet high in leguminous fibre (beans, peas and lentils) should be positively encouraged.
  - The use of a low-fat diet may reduce cardiovascular risk.
  - In the long term the aim is that 50–60% of the dietary energy should be in the form of carbohdrate. The bulk of this carbohydrate should come from starches, not sugars. A small quantity of sugar can, however, be included in the diet, provided it is consumed as part of a diet which is low in fat and high in sources of natural dietary fibre.
  - Overweight patients should be encouraged to reduce their total calorie intake and to aim for ideal body weight.
- The diet needs must be individually tailored and regularly updated to take into account the patient's age, weight, work, hobbies and ethnic preferences. This is where advice from a professional dietitian is invaluable.
- Referral to the dietitian on the diet request card should be clearly written, and should give full patient details, including full address and name of family practitioner, district nurse (if known), current treatment and especially the reason for referral. An indication of the degree of urgency of the request is important, and clear instructions of the best time and method to communicate with the patient (e.g. daytime telephone number, etc.) should also be noted.
- The referral form is also used by the dietitians as their record card, and is filed in the case notes for future reference.

CHIROPODY
REQUEST CARD AND RECORD

(IDENTIFICATION LABEL)

UNIT NO. 123456

SURNAME AHOLIC

FIRST NAME(S) CHOC

ADDRESS 2, SUGAR LUMPS
SWEETOOTH

DOB

CLINIC Diabetic Clinic

CONSULTANT/GP Dr. Hyde

PATIENT MEDICATION Sugar free diet and Tolbutamide

DIAGNOSIS, CLINICAL DETAILS

Diabetes diagnosed 1993. Good foot pulses. Sensory diminution at toe tips.

Clawed toes. High plantar arch. Callus under ball of foot.

DATE 10.2.95 M.R. Hyde

REPORT DATES			

Chiropodist referral form

- The chiropodist is a key member of the team providing care for people with diabetes, and plays a very important role in the treatment of the patient with foot problems and in the education of the patient, the immediate family and other carers.
- The chiropodist also plays an important role in the education of the other diabetes team members, and in increasing and maintaining a high degree of awareness of the nature of diabetic foot problems.
- Another benefit of regular chiropody attendance for the person with diabetes is that it ensures regular inspection of the feet (and the footwear) by an experienced clinical observer, and each visit to the chiropodist gives an opportunity for reinforcing diabetic footcare advice.
- All people with diabetes who have evidence of neuropathy, foot deformity, peripheral vascular insufficiency or callus formation are at increased risk of foot ulceration and should be referred to a chiropodist.
- It is important that the chiropody referral form or request card is completed accurately and that it gives full details of the type of diabetes, nature of medication and an indication of the nature of the identified foot problem, as well as brief comments on the state of the peripheral vasculature and the presence or absence of neuropathic signs or symptoms.
- The chiropody referral form or request card can be used as the chiropodist's clinical record and filed in the patient's case notes for future reference.

Computerised shared care facilitation in diabetes

- A structured system of care, shared between hospital and primary care teams, probably represents the best setting for the effective management of the majority of people with diabetes.
- The recording and transmission of accurate information is an essential requirement for the success of such a system of shared care. Information technology offers advantages over manual records in facilitating data gathering and storage, and in supporting accurate, timely communication within the diabetes team and between hospitals and primary care.
- A computerised register of the population with diabetes can be established in a district and utilised to support regular review by means of computer-generated call and recall, and follow-up of non-attenders.
- Computerised data gathering can facilitate regular audit of the standard of diabetes care in a district.
- A computerised clinic record system can be used to complement standard paper records and can incorporate a report/letter-writing facility for production of automated clinic reports and discharge letters.
- Computer programs can be designed which aid clinical decision making relating to differential diagnoses and/or therapy decisions in diabetes.
- Computerised storage of digitally acquired images such as retinal photographs can help in monitoring progression of disease as well as allowing transmission of images for distant specialist evaluation and diagnosis.
- Computer systems should be flexible, easy to use in a clinic setting and should not interfere with the establishment of good clinical rapport between doctor or nurse and patient.
- Watertight systems must be built in to guarantee absolute confidentiality of sensitive patient information.

Local diabetes service advisory groups

- In an attempt to meet the targets set out in the St Vincent Declaration, some countries have promoted the idea of establishing local diabetes service advisory groups (LDSAGs).
- LDSAGs contribute to the formation of a comprehensive local strategy for diabetes management, and help to improve local care for people with diabetes by advising upon and monitoring the health care and social services available for people with diabetes, and by advising on improvements (clinical and administrative) to provide a high-quality service which will meet their needs and wishes.
- Membership of LDSAGs should include representatives of specialist and primary care health professionals and people with diabetes and their carers, all working together with representatives of the managers of the service and the purchasers or commissioners of these services.
- LDSAGs should advise on national and local guidelines on diabetes services, on new scientific developments and advances in clinical care, and on the implementation of the recommendations of the St Vincent Declaration.
- LDSAGs should be concerned with the following:
  - developing a local strategy for diabetes care and prevention taking into account the needs of the local population of people with diabetes, setting specific objectives and targets to improve the health of people with diabetes;
  - advising on the development of a specification of the services required to meet the needs of local people with diabetes which would take into account the views of service users; and
  - developing systems to facilitate the achievement of the targets set and provision of patient satisfaction.

Appendices

The choice of insulin: by duration of action

This whole area is a minefield for the uninitiated and unwary (and even for the expert!).

- Insulins can be categorised according to their duration of action, which is determined by the type of additive to which the insulin is bound.
  - *Soluble insulin* (sometimes known as 'neutral insulin' because most preparations are buffered to neutral pH to offset the irritant effect of the acid pH of early insulin extracts). Peak action following subcutaneous injection is usually within 1 hour and lasts 2–4 hours then gradually declines over the next 4 hours—a short-acting insulin which needs to be injected more than once a day. In the United States this insulin is known as 'regular' insulin.
  - *Isophane insulin* (sometimes known as 'neutral protamine Hagedorn' (NPH) because it is at neutral pH, is bound to protamine—a protein derived from fish semen—in order to delay the insulin absorbtion from the subcutis, and was first prepared in the Hagedorn laboratories in Germany). Peak action following subcutaneous injection occurs in about 2–4 hours, lasts a further 2–4 hours then gradually declines over the next 6–8 hours—a medium-acting insulin which can sometimes be used once a day but usually needs to be injected more than once a day.
  - *Lente insulins* (also known as 'insulin zinc suspensions' (IZS) because they consist of suspensions of amorphous and/or crystalline insulin suspended with a suitable zinc salt to which the insulin adsorbs. This serves to delay the insulin absorbtion from the subcutis.) The onset and duration of action of these insulins depends on the nature of the insulin suspension. *Semilente insulin* is an insulin zinc suspension containing insulin in the amorphous form only. Peak action following subcutaneous injection occurs in about 1 hour, lasts 2–6 hours then gradually declines over the next 4–6 hours—a medium-acting insulin which needs to be injected more than once a day. *Lente insulin* is an insulin zinc suspension containing insulin in both amorphous and crystalline

forms. Peak action following subcutaneous injection occurs in about 2–4 hours, lasts 6–12 hours then gradually declines over the next 8–10 hours—a medium- to long-acting insulin which can be suitable for injection once or twice a day. *Ultralente insulin* is an insulin zinc suspension containing insulin in the crystalline form only. Peak action following subcutaneous injection occurs in about 4–6 hours, lasts 8–12 hours then gradually declines over the next 8–12 hours—a long-acting insulin which is suitable for injection once a day.

- *Protamine zinc insulin* ((PZI)—insulin suspended in a mixture with both zinc and protamine so that its absorbtion from the subcutis is significantly delayed) is seldom used nowadays because its profile of action is very variable especially if mixed in the syringe with soluble insulin which adsorbs to surplus protamine to an unpredictable extent. Peak action following subcutaneous injection occurs in about 4–6 hours, lasts 8–12 hours then gradually declines over the next 6–10 hours—a long-acting insulin which is suitable for injection once a day.
- *Biphasic insulin preparations.* These are ready-made fixed mixtures of rapid-acting (soluble) insulin and intermediate-acting (usually isophane) insulin which are suitable for twice-daily injection. They are manufactured in varying fixed proportions (from 10:90% to 50:50%) which gives a flexibility of actions which can be tailored to individuals' needs.

The choice of insulin: by species of origin or molecular configuration

- Insulin was first extracted in Toronto in 1921 by Frederick Banting and Charles Best by a process of alcohol extraction from crude islet preparations extracted from the pancreases of dogs. Subsequent thoughts about commercial insulin extraction included consideration of the possibility of using pancreatic extract from fish pancreases—a potentially useful byproduct of the lucrative Canadian salmon industry.
- The first successful commercial extraction of insulin by the Eli Lilly company in the United States relied on a supply of beef pancreases from the abattoirs of the American mid-west. For many years insulin of bovine origin was the only available injectable insulin for therapeutic use in humans.
- When the patent for insulin production for European use was passed to the Novo company in Denmark, the possibility of using the Danish bacon industry as a source of pig pancreases was exploited, so porcine insulin became available for human use.
- In the 1960s and 1970s the refinement of chemical techniques and the development of genetic engineering techniques for modification and/or synthesis of complex molecules allowed the commercial production of insulin which was chemically identical to insulin of human origin, thus reducing the dependence of the insulin manufacturers on the meat industry and potentially decreasing the antigenicity of the insulin.
  - *Beef insulin.* Differs from human insulin by three amino acids. Still very widely used in some Third-World countries, but currently falling in popularity in western countries. Potentially more immunogenic than human insulin and this may be important in the causation of some rare cases of insulin allergy or antibody-mediated insulin resistance. Injection-site lipoatrophy is also a manifestation of immune response which occurs much more often with insulin of bovine origin than with porcine insulin, and hardly at all with human insulin.
  - *Pork insulin.* Differs from human insulin by one amino acid. A very suitable substitute for human insulin for patients who

have problems with hypoglycaemic unawareness or other reasons for not going onto human insulin.

- *Human insulin.* Many theoretical advantages over insulins of animal origin, but these are not always borne out in clinical practice. A wider range of preparations are available than of animal insulins. Manufacture of human insulin by genetic engineering takes away the reliance on animal tissues as a source of insulin, so getting away from the potential for transmission of infections such as bovine spongiform encephalopathy (although this has not been shown to be a real danger). Until recently, only human insulins have been available in forms suitable for giving through pen injection devices.
- *Insulin analogues.* Further modification of the insulin molecule by recombinant genetic engineering techniques has led to the potential for commercial production of insulin analogues. These have the same biological activity as native insulin but have different profiles of action and the potential for a greater range of therapeutic options offering an increased flexibility of insulin regimens.

The choice of oral hypoglycaemic drugs: sulphonylurea drugs

- These drugs (chemically related to sulphonamide antimicrobials) work mainly by augmenting pancreatic insulin production. Although in long-term use they also have a slight extra-pancreatic action, probably at the level of tissue insulin receptors, they can only really be effective in patients who have some residual pancreatic beta-cell function. They are therefore of no value on their own in patients with Type 1 diabetes. As beta-cell function often gradually fails even in patients with Type 2 diabetes, their effectiveness may diminish with time even in these patients, resulting in a need for ever-increasing doses up to the maximum effective dose. This may be followed by the need for addition of a second and even a third oral hypoglycaemic agent, and finally a need to consider starting insulin therapy. This may occur even in patients who have been maintained on tablets for years.
- Glibenclamide and chlorpropamide have been available for many years and are still widely used. Both are long acting and need to be given only once a day, before the first meal of the day. Tolazamide and acetohexamide are two other long-acting drugs, which are less frequently used in the United Kingdom.
- Tolbutamide, which has also been available for many years, is a shorter-acting drug which is given two or three times a day, before each main meal.
- Newer agents such as gliclazide, glibornuride and glipizide probably offer no clinically significant further benefit over the older drugs, except that they may be useful alternatives in patients with renal dysfunction, as they are excreted in bile, not through the kidneys.
- All sulphonylureas can cause weight gain and are therefore most useful in patients who are less than 20% above their ideal body weight.
- Side-effects are relatively mild and uncommon and include gastrointestinal upset, headache and allergic skin rashes. Chlorpropamide rarely causes intra-hepatic cholestasis with jaundice, and this has also been reported with some of the other sulphonylureas. Blood dyscrasias and severe exfoliative

dermatoses are very rare manifestations of sensitivity reactions to these drugs.

- Chlorpropamide may cause facial flushing in patients after drinking alcohol. There was once a great deal of research directed towards this phenomenon, which was thought to be a marker for a particular inherited trait in some people with diabetes which might have been associated with relative protection from diabetic tissue damage. However, this has now been shown not to be the case, and chlorpropamide–alcohol flushing is now recognised simply as a variable and probably dose-dependent side-effect.
- All sulphonylureas should be started in the lowest possible recommended dose because they are capable of producing severe hypoglycaemia especially in elderly patients who might be prone to erratic eating or who might have some hepatic or renal dysfunction. Although hypoglycaemia may often be obvious, sometimes patients present with atypical symptoms such as dizziness, headaches, transient lateralised weakness, forgetfulness and confusion. These symptoms may be wrongly ascribed to cerebrovascular disease or a dementing process, whereas they may respond dramatically to reduction in the dose of the sulphonylurea. Hypoglycaemia is commonest in patients taking the longer-acting agents. Glibenclamide can produce hypoglycaemia in up to 20% of patients, and this can be severe and life-threatening.
- If patients remain poorly controlled despite maximum tolerated doses of a sulphonylurea drug, then metformin and/or acarbose can be introduced and the dosage increased until acceptable glycaemic control is achieved. If blood sugars remain high despite maximal doses of a combination of oral agents (tablet failure) then introduction of insulin therapy must be considered.

The choice of oral hypoglycaemic drugs: biguanides

- Metformin is currently the only available biguanide, since the related drug phenformin was withdrawn because its use was associated with an unacceptably high risk of causing the potentially serious complication of lactic acidosis. The risk is much lower with metformin, although it is not entirely free of this hazard. For this reason metformin should not be used in patients with renal dysfunction, and should only be used cautiously in patients with hepatic dysfunction and other conditions which might increase the tendency to build-up of tissue lactic acid levels, such as cardiac failure, severe tissue trauma or sepsis, dehydration and alcohol dependence.
- Metformin has to be taken in two or three doses throughout the day, usually with or immediately after the main meals.
- Like sulphonylurea drugs, metformin only works in the presence of endogenous insulin and therefore can only really be effective in patients who have some residual pancreatic beta-cell function. It is therefore of no value on its own in patients with Type 1 diabetes.
- Unlike sulphonylurea drugs, metformin does not work by augmenting pancreatic insulin production but by increasing the effectiveness of insulin action at the periphery. It does this in part by reducing hepatic gluconeogenesis, and in part by increasing peripheral tissue uptake of glucose.
- Metformin has a slight anorectic effect and therefore is not usually associated with the problem of unacceptable weight gain which can limit the effectiveness of the sulphonylurea drugs. For this reason metformin is most useful in patients who are more than 20% above their ideal body weight and who have failed to achieve normoglycaemia with dietary measures alone.
- Metformin does not exert a hypoglycaemic effect in non-diabetic subjects unless taken in overdosage, and when used as a sole agent in patients with diabetes the risk of causing severe hypoglycaemia is negligible in conventional doses. Severe hypoglycaemia due to concomitant sulphonylurea therapy may be exacerbated by metformin and it may be necessary to

consider reducing the dose of sulphonylurea when metformin is added to therapy.

- Metformin causes gastrointestinal side-effects in up to 20% of patients. These are sometimes transitory and the patient may learn to tolerate the effects (which may contribute to the beneficial anorectic effect mentioned above!). However, in many patients the unpleasant side-effects of nausea, abdominal pains and/or diarrhoea may persist and prove intolerable, necessitating the cessation of the drug.
- If patients remain poorly controlled despite maximum tolerated doses of metformin then a sulphonylurea drug and/or acarbose can be introduced, and the dosages increased until acceptable glycaemic control is achieved. If blood sugars remain high despite maximally tolerated doses of a combination of oral hypoglycaemic agents (tablet failure) then introduction of insulin therapy must be considered.

The choice of oral hypoglycaemic drugs: alpha-1-glucosidase inhibitors

- Acarbose is the only member of this group of agents available at the time of writing, although another alpha-1-glucosidase inhibitor, miglitol, is undergoing trials, and it is likely that other related agents are also in development.
- Acarbose is a competitive antagonist of the enzyme alpha-1-glucosidase which is located on the brush border of the villi of the small intestine. This enzyme is responsible for breaking down dietary disaccharides and polysaccharides to their monosaccharide components, mainly glucose, for absorbtion through the intestinal wall into the bloodstream. Thus, by blocking this action acarbose has the effect of significantly reducing the amount of glucose absorbed into the blood from the intestine after meals and significantly reduces post-prandial glycaemic excursions.
- Acarbose can be used as first-line oral hypoglycaemic therapy in patients with Type 2 diabetes whose diabetes has not come under control on dietary measures alone.
- Acarbose can also be used in conjunction with sulphonylurea drugs and/or metformin when these agents on their own or in combination have failed to bring about satisfactory glycaemic control.
- Because acarbose inhibits the breakdown of dietary disaccharides and polysaccharides in the small intestine, these compounds pass relatively unaltered down into the caecum and large intestine. Here they provide substrate for fermentation by intestinal bacteria. This sometimes leads to significant intestinal gas production which is responsible for the most commonly reported side-effect of this agent, namely abdominal distension and subsequent discomfort with excess flatulence and looseness of bowel motion, sometimes with frank diarrhoea. These side-effects may be reduced by a very gradual introduction of the drug, initially in a once-daily dose of 50 mg with the first mouthful of the first meal of the day, increasing to a twice-daily dosage only after 3–4 weeks, and making further small incremental doses at similar intervals up to the maximum required or tolerated dose, whichever is the earliest.

- The problems of flatulence and abdominal discomfort with disturbance of bowel habit are much more likely to occur in people who do not comply strictly with instructions to avoid sugar, because eating sucrose when taking acarbose will significantly increase the amount of disaccharide which will pass through to the colon for bacterial fermentation.
- Acarbose taken on its own will not cause significant symptomatic hypoglycaemia. However, when it is used in combination with sulphonylureas it can increase the risk of sulphonylurea-related hypoglycaemic symptoms occurring. For this reason it may be prudent to consider reducing the dose of sulphonylurea drugs when introducing adjunctive acarbose treatment.
- If sulphonylurea-related hypoglycaemia does occur in a patient who is also taking acarbose then it is important to remember that it will not be corrected by giving sugar orally, because acarbose will inhibit the breakdown of sucrose into glucose and maltose in the small intestine, so the blood glucose will not rise significantly in response to sugar. Instead, oral glucose must be given to correct hypoglycaemia in patients taking acarbose in addition to sulphonylurea drugs.
- Acarbose can rarely cause reversible disturbance of biochemical tests of liver function, but has no other significant systemic adverse effects.

The choice of oral hypoglycaemic drugs: thiazolidinediones—insulin action enhancers

- The pathophysiology of Type 2 diabetes is characterised by defects in both insulin secretion and insulin resistance. Insulin resistance is present in virtually all patients with Type 2 diabetes and is apparent early in the course of the disease.
- Insulin resistance is considered important in the development and progression of Type 2 diabetes, causing premature beta-cell exhaustion because of the demands on insulin secretion. There is also evidence that insulin resistance is central to the cardiovascular and microvascular consequences of Type 2 diabetes.
- Troglitazone was the first commercially available member of the thiazolidinediones, a new class of oral antidiabetic agents, known as insulin action enhancers.
- Troglitazone appeared to target insulin resistance, by re-sensitising the body to the action of its own insulin. It enhanced glucose utilisation by increasing glycogen synthetase activity thus increasing muscle uptake of glucose. It also reduced hepatic glucose production by reducing gluconeogenesis.
- Troglitazone appeared to have a beneficial effect on cardiovascular risk factors—decreasing insulin levels, raising HDL cholesterol and reducing triglycerides. Troglitazone seemed to affect the fundamental abnormalities which confer increased risk of cardiovascular disease in the insulin resistance syndrome and in Type 2 diabetes.
- The use of troglitazone was, however, found to be associated with hepatocellular damage in some people, especially those who had taken it for more than 3 months. This damage appeared to be irreversible and associated with fatal liver necrosis in some cases. Troglitazone was therefore withdrawn from use in the United Kingdom. Work is currently underway to try and develop safer insulin action enhancing drugs.

Further reading

Boulton AJM (ed). *Diabetic Neuropathy*. Carnforth: Marius Press, 1996.

Boulton AJM, Connor H, Cavanagh PR (eds). *The Foot in Diabetes*, 2nd edn. Chichester: John Wiley & Sons, 1994.

The Diabetes Control and Complications Trial Research Group. The effect of intensive treatment of diabetes on the development and progression of long-term complications in insulin-dependent diabetes mellitus. *N Engl J Med* 1993; **329**: 977–86.

Finucane P, Sinclair AJ (eds). *Diabetes in Old Age*. Chichester: John Wiley & Sons, 1995.

Kritzinger EE, Taylor KG. *Diabetic Eye Disease: An Illustrated Guide to Diagnosis and Management*. Lancaster: MTP Press Ltd, 1984.

Pickup JC, Williams G (eds). *Textbook of Diabetes*, 2nd edn. Oxford: Blackwell Science, 1997.

Reaven GM. Role of insulin resistance in human disease. *Diabetes* 1988; **37**: 1595–607.

Spiro JG, Watts GF. The skin in diabetes. *Practical Diabetes* 1986; **3**: 196–9.

UK Prospective Diabetes Study Group. Overview of 6 years' therapy of type 2 diabetes: a progressive disease. *Diabetes* 1995; **44**: 1249–58.

World Health Organization Europe and European Region of International Diabetes Federation. *The St Vincent Declaration*. Copenhagen: WHO Europe and the European Region of IDF, 1989.

Index

[redacted]